Practical Infection Control

A Health Care Professional and

Community Resource Guide

Nevio Cimolai
Debra J. Cimolai

Populus Productions and Publishing Ltd., British Columbia, Canada, 2012

ISBN: 978 0 9866421 9 7

Published by Populus Productions and Publishing Ltd.

Current printing: First Edition

The authors dedicate this book to the living memories of Tomas, Marnai, and Francis Cimolai.

Cover: Populus Productions and Publishing Ltd., 2012.

Cimolai, N., Cimolai, D. Practical Infection Control: A Health Care Professional and Community Resource Guide. British Columbia, Canada:Populus Productions and Publishing Ltd., 2012.

Foreword

The collaboration of health care professionals in an integrated community and hospital environment is as important today as it ever has been. Yet the current changes in the health care climate have forced both the medical and non-medical communities to heighten their awareness of this truth and to practically realize the potential. In preparing this textbook, we were comfortable that our experience in primary and tertiary hospital care, community nursing and general practice, public health, university academics, administration and teaching, not to mention the experience of everyday family life and occupation, would provide us with the necessary skills that were required to design a text for the broad category of the health care professional. We also realized during the preparation of the text that, given the sophistication of everyday society as it has evolved to this first printing, there was considerable relevance to the general community.

We did not attempt to recreate a detailed manual that would strictly define policy and procedure for hospital infection control. There are several medical texts which have exactly carried out such function. Rather, we propose that the need is to reach the primary caregiver in whatever role that individual maintains. The general knowledge base in this area, as well as the skills which arise, are broadly applicable. Whereas there may be a tendency from the pure medical and nursing perspective to reduce much of the scope to numbers and statistics, we have strived to provide the reader with context, perspective, learning, experience, and perhaps some humility.

Health care professionals are a diverse group of individuals. Although we could not cater all of the content to every specific individual, we have written this book with the intent of ensuring that there is something relevant for everyone with more or less emphasis. Even those less schooled in health care will grasp the salient features of infection control, for they too are critical to realizing a practical infection control both in medical institutions and in the community.

Infection control in its broadest sense is of relevance to us all. Knowingly or not, we apply its principles in our clinics, in our hospitals, and in our everyday lives. The word "hygiene" might come back into an equivalent and popular use if only we realized that its origin describes the preservation of health and therefore indirectly the prevention of transmission for infectious agents. We hope that you will not only enjoy the format and knowledge base, but also practically realize useful and effective translation into everyday caregiving and living.

Nevio and Debra Cimolai

Proviso

Medicine and the science of infection are ever-changing fields. Whereas we have attempted to bring the reader up-to-date in regards to infection control, there may be examples where the progress has leaped beyond our publication. The reader is advised to consult their local experts and to examine contemporary medical literature when problems arise and when common sense does not apparently prevail.

The readers must accept the application of infection control practice at their own risk. We cannot assure positive outcome when the techniques we describe or the information we provide are implemented, nor do we make any such representation in whole or in part. Neither the authors nor publisher can be held responsible, or liable, in any way for the audience's use or interpretation of this guide's information.

"A man's own observation, what he finds good of and what he finds hurt of, is the best physic to preserve health."

Francis Bacon
Essays, Of Regimen of Health, 1625

Table of Contents

Foreward
Proviso

"All interest in disease and death is only another expression of interest in life."

Thomas Mann
The Magic Mountain, 1924

I. The Roots of Infection Control

What is Infection Control ?

In broad terms, **Infection Control** is concerned with the prevention of transmission of infection to a human (Figure 1). The agent which is being transmitted is generally a member of the complex microbial world, and there are conceivably many germs, either simple or complex, which can cause infection. For some individuals, acquisition of the microbe will subsequently lead to infection whether mild or severe. For others, the acquisition may lead only to a transient or permanent carriage without subsequent infection; this carriage may be termed **colonization**, and the person may only serve as an intermediary in the chain of events. All humans may be implicated therefore in the spread of germs whether or not they are infected. The ability to cause infection is ultimately determined by the human-microbial interaction which is dependent on a number of characteristics of each.

The source for the transmitted microbe will often be another human who is shedding the viable infectious germ during an active infection or while

Figure 1. The foundations of infection control.

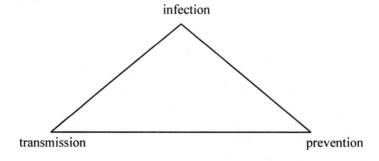

colonized. In addition to human sources, other mammalian species and many other members of the animal kingdom can act as the source depending on the specific micro-organism. Outside of the latter foci, almost any other facet of nature, whether plant, water, or earth, may serve to harbour a particular microbe which at sometime will be capable of causing infection when it reaches the susceptible individual. These sources are often called **reservoirs** of infection, and they may be permanent or temporary.

The actual transfer of the infectious agent to a human can be accomplished in several ways. Direct contact (including ingestion) is an obvious route and according to many, the most important mechanism. Transmission by air (aerosol) or by a passive intermediary (**vector**) are also of practical concern.

If we understand who may suffer from infection, where the infectious agent comes from, and how the transfer can occur, it will be obvious how prevention can be facilitated. These are the fundamentals of infection control no matter how complex the infection or how large the outbreak. The tools of infection control may therefore be as simple as handwashing or quarantine of the infected or colonized patient. They may be as complex as an exploitation of the new technologies to create a vaccine or to synthesize a new antibiotic, the latter which will either treat an infection appropriately or provide prevention (**prophylaxis**). In days of yore, infection control on a practical basis was embodied by the word "hygiene". Indeed, institutes of hygiene were so named historically in part to further the knowledge of infection control in both hospital and community; these have now given way to our public health bodies and academic colleges.

More strictly speaking, however, the term infection control is often used by health care professionals to describe the efforts of a hospital infection containment, monitoring, and prevention program. Hospital-acquired infections (**nosocomial**) have great implications given the pooling of sick individuals and their particular susceptibility. We must recognize, however, that the true impact of infection control issues extends well beyond the hospital environment even though, historically, we have often thought of infection control merely as a hospital issue.

A Rich History

Among health care professionals, an understanding of our past is no less important than in other disciplines for the purposes of understanding our present and for creating our future. Many of our contemporary infection control dilemmas are solved by simple maneuvers which have had their origin in decades if not centuries past, and many solutions count on simply re-inventing the wheel or at least recognizing that the wheel was built so in the past for good reason. Though many aspects of medicine have a rich and colorful history, arguably very few have as much historical complexity as infection and its control.

It is difficult to know when the concepts of infection and its spread were practically realized, but concerns for transmissible agents of disease must have been apparent well before civilization if not only because of obvious food-borne sicknesses. There are many highlights which illustrate humanity's growth in the understanding of infection and its spread. We can only hope to illustrate examples of this growth since the individual contributions have been numerous (Table 1). For centuries, it was evident to many that food preservation could be accomplished by salting, drying, or fermentation (i.e., alcohol-producing such as wine, or acid-producing such as yoghurt) even though it was not apparent that food spoilage was caused by microbes. The preservation of body tissue by embalming in ancient Egypt was unknowingly an exercise of hindering microbial growth. The concept of an infectious disease or the spread of contagion must

Table 1. Milestones in the history of infection and infection control.

~100-200 AD	Galen - theories of transmission Thucydides - acquired immunity
1500s	Fracastorius - epidemiology
1700s	Van Leeuwenhoek - microscopy Spallanzani - sterility Martens/Hunter - contagion Jenner - vaccination
1800s	Pasteur - pasteurization; germ theory Tyndall - spores
1900s	Snow - outbreak investigation Holmes/Semmelweis - handwashing Lister - antisepsis Koch - laboratory bacteriology Loeffler/Frosch - laboratory virology Von Behring/Kitasato - antisera
20th century	Fleming/Domagk - antibiotics
21th century	many!!! - burgeoning of molecular biology

have been recognized in pre-Biblical times as it was obvious in many circumstances that contact with an ill person, or with objects that the ill person had contaminated, could lead to subsequent disease. The great surgeon and physician **Galen** had coined the term gonorrhea meaning "flow of seed" in describing the seeding of infection from one individual to the sexual contact. Whereas the ancient Hebrews may have viewed infection, or pestilence, as a punishment from above, they nevertheless had a sense of infection control by isolating lepers. It is quite possible that their dietary limitations for shellfish and pork were unknowingly more out of concern for illnesses (especially infection) after consumption than for any other reason. Concepts of immunity were also apparent - **Thucydides** recognized that individuals who recovered from certain illnesses were incapable of suffering from the same disease again. Indeed, it was those who had become ill and recovered that were unafraid of caring for the sick and dying - for good reason: an acquired immunity.

As one might imagine, numerous individuals at various times had put forward theories relating to infection and its control which scientifically were sensible and which would subsequently prove to be correct. Yet there was more that could not be explained, and progress in the science must have been difficult if not only due to the many, then unknown, transmissible diseases and their variations. Superstitions, mysticism, and lack of knowledge were all to cloud any possible gain. What subsequently evolved, however, was the "germ theory". Soon after, knowledge of transmissible agents, prevention of transmission, and protective immunity would emerge.

In the sixteenth century, **Fracastorius** published his *"De Contagione"* which some propose was the beginning of the science of epidemiology (the study of factors which determine the distribution and frequency of disease). Like Galen in his description of gonorrhea, Fracastorius believed that disease was spread by "seminaria" or seeds. This spread was again recognized as either person-to-person or through inanimate objects. **Van Leeuwenhoek** in the eighteenth century initiated the theory of germs in part when he developed the microscope sufficiently to be able to see what were microbes. **Spallanzani** observed that a meat broth would remain unspoiled indefinitely if it was boiled and sealed, but **Pasteur** would subsequently be credited with the germ theory in the next century.

In the eighteenth century, **Martens** promoted a theory that tuberculosis (then called consumption) was contagious. **Hunter** furthered the belief in contagiousness by transmitting gonorrhea to himself from the infected genital secretions of a patient. Little did Hunter know that we would also contact syphilis from these same secretions! **Jenner**'s work on smallpox vaccination demonstrated that infection could be spread by direct contact and an infection could modify immunity.

The nineteenth century yielded key discoveries that would dramatically and permanently change the science. **Pasteur** essentially confirmed the germ theory and dispelled the popular belief that germs arose do novo (theory of spontaneous generation). The use of heat treatment to eradicate microbes (hence *pasteur*ization) became firmly entrenched. A mild set-back was experienced when **Tyndall** discovered that heat-resistant bacteria were capable of eluding Pasteur's techniques. **Cohn**, however, was subsequently able to explain heat resistance by the presence of spores (sessile, environment resistant forms) in some bacteria. Pasteur's theory would survive! Also in this century, **Snow**'s masterful detective work showed that a cholera epidemic could be traced to a single water pump which had spread disease from a water supply that was contaminated with fecal waste. The transmissible nature of infection was then furthered when **Villemin** was able to infect animals with human tuberculosis. **Holmes** and **Semmelweis**, who were working independently on different continents, simultaneously illustrated that handwashing was a simple yet effective method of preventing spread - obstetricians were directly responsible for perinatal and post-partum infections by examining the genital tracts of patients one after another without washing their (bare) hands!

Beyond the value of handwashing, **Lister** illustrated the benefits of disinfection. He introduced the concept of antiseptics in surgery by showing how a topical germicide could reduce the frequency of post-operative wound infections. By 1877, **Koch** had isolated a human pathogen, *Bacillus anthracis* (the cause of anthrax), in the laboratory. Indeed most of the human pathogenic bacteria were cultivated in the laboratory over the subsequent twenty years. **Loeffler** and **Frosch** unknowingly began modern virology (the study of viruses) when they demonstrated that cell-free filtrates could transmit foot and mouth disease among cattle.

Given that the germ theory and relevant specific agents were now recognized, and that transmission was possible, the two key areas of immunology (the study of the body's resistance) and drug therapy would inevitably emerge. In these regards, **von Behring** and **Kitasato** realized the ability of sera (a blood fraction) to have tetanus toxin neutralizing ability; immunity to microbial agents was possible. **Fleming**'s recognition that a compound from the *Penicillium* mold (penicillin) could inhibit some bacteria, and **Domagk**'s creation of precursors to sulpha drugs would lead to a new era in the battle between pathogen and human.

The finding of new microbial pathogens, the molecular biology revolution and its new tools, an expanding spectrum of antibiotics, and the development of new vaccines have tremendously changed the way we think about and then manage infection. The rudimentary foundations for infection control nevertheless have remained.

Why Is Infection Control Important ?

The impact of infection on our everyday lives is quite evident, whether on the basis of the infections which we personally suffer or from the many issues relating to infection that we hear about in the lay press. The absolute numbers of, the morbidity from, and the mortality from infection that is spread are simply impressive.

There are many examples which illustrate how infection control is important. If one only examines the impact of hospital-acquired (nosocomial) infection for in-patients, estimates have varied in the $500 to $4000 U.S. range for the average cost of such an infection. Whereas the estimate reflects an average, there are patients whose outcome of hospital care may be dramatically affected. For example, hospital-acquired infection is not an uncommon cause of death. The following clinical vignettes exemplify the potential consequences:

> *An eight week old female was born cyanotic and was found to have congenital heart disease which would require cardiovascular surgery. Due to intermittent respiratory problems which were associated with the heart dysfunction, the infant was admitted to hospital for assessment two days prior to the elective surgery. On the fourth hospital day, intended for surgery, the child had manifestations of an upper respiratory infection which quickly progressed into a bronchiolitis.* Respiratory syncytial virus *was determined as the cause; exactly the same virus coincidentally found to be causing a mild respiratory illness in a two week old room mate who was admitted for apnea on the same day of admission as the former. Surgery for the eight week old child was delayed for seven days. After surgery, the child developed a superficial wound infection secondary to* Staphylococcus aureus *which required antimicrobial treatment. As a result of the antibiotic therapy, however, the child developed antibiotic-associated diarrhea secondary to* Clostridium difficile. *The patient*

was discharged well after twenty-eight days of hospital care.

An eighty year old gentleman underwent an elective out-patient prostatectomy. He returned to his physician two days later with complaints of fever, chills, and a general feeling of unwell. He was found to have low blood pressure and was admitted to hospital for suspected infection. The man suffered a stormy course. He developed shock and respiratory distress, hence requiring mechanical ventilation. He was oliguric and needed pharmacological support for his circulation. Escherichia coli *urinary infection and blood-borne infection were established. The bacterium was subsequently found to be resistant to the antibiotic regimen which was initially chosen, and a new regimen was instituted. The individual was being weaned from ventilatory support when on day seven of the admission, he developed a pneumonia secondary to* Pseudomonas aeruginosa. *Three other chronically ventilated patients in the intensive care unit had yielded the same bacterium in tracheal secretions. The antibiotic regimen was again changed, but the respiratory infection prolonged his ventilation requirements. During this time, the patient was catheterized for urinary incontinence. As a consequence, he developed another urinary tract infection. Again the bacterium entered the bloodstream, and the patient eventually succumbed. This time, the bacterium was multiply resistant to most antibiotics. A similar strain of organism had been infecting the bladder of another intensively cared-for patient who was catheterized and who received multiple antibiotics in the process of treating complications from a motor vehicle accident.*

These nosocomial infections, although dramatic, serve to highlight several key points. The direct costs of acquired infection are many. These may range from increased requirements for nursing staff, increased use of consumables (e.g., dressings, microbial culture, ventilator tubing, antibiotics, to name a few), physician time, support from many other hospital professionals, among others. From a conservative estimate, the daily cost of an additional hospital day in most western hospitals is approximately $1000 U.S., and this is significantly increased if these are intensive care unit days. The indirect costs are also considerable and less often thought of. How can one express the cost of additional suffering, or for that matter, a death? How to measure the costs of negatively impacting a family and caregivers? The pooling of patients in hospital, a milieu where other ill patients that may have infection reside, is in itself a major risk factor for a transmissible disease. A medical or surgical intervention, which often takes place in hospitals, can be a major risk factor for subsequent infection - the use of antibiotics or surgery to deal with a hospital infection may be absolutely required but may in themselves cause the patient to become susceptible to a new nosocomial infection! Perhaps seemingly less costly on a per diem basis, it is nevertheless possible that infections acquired in long-term care, ambulatory clinics, and home care are as impactful regarding patient morbidity and mortality.

What seems a brief incident or one which involves only one infected patient may appear initially minor, but, given the particular circumstances, may prove to be onerous and impactful. Examples of such could be many but consider only the following: 1) chicken pox in a hospital cancer ward where immune compromised individuals may be at risk for systemic disease, 2) a pregnant female with active rubella who visits her obstetrician in the midst of a waiting room which is full with other gravid ladies, 3) human plague in a small community in an underdeveloped country where the knowledge of communicability and the availability of treatment and quarantine facilities are limited, 4) active pulmonary tuberculosis in an open general hospital ward, and 5) meningococcal meningitis in a child who schools in a large classroom. The subsequent cascade of real concerns, anxiety, and actual work are sufficient to necessitate considerable effort towards dealing with the issue at hand and then towards ensuring prevention for the next time.

Is infection control really worth it? For all of the activities that occur both within the community and the medical care facility, this question is a common one from administrators, government, and the public. On a generic basis, the obvious answer is a resounding "yes"! One only needs to go back in time to see what it was "really like" to appreciate the impact of infection control measures. How dangerous was surgery when antisepsis was not understood and antibiotics were not available? How many people died of smallpox, polio, diphtheria, and neonatal tetanus prior to the production of effective vaccines? (Table 2; see also Chapter XVII) Apart from the effect of war, how would infections have changed the history of the world in the modern era if current efforts in infection control were not had? It is evidently not a source for controversy when one appreciates the impact of infection control on an all or none basis. If there is to be any debate about the relevance of infection control, it can only be with respect to micro-management issues and with concerns that are very pointed.

Table 2. Examples of historically important epidemics of contagion.

1300s	plague in Europe
1600-1700s	smallpox in North America
1800s	tuberculosis in Europe cholera in India and neighbouring countries polio epidemics worldwide
1918-1919	worldwide influenza pandemic
1940s	meningococcal outbreaks during World War 2 relapsing fever during World War 2
Pre-vaccine era	measles, mumps, rubella, whooping cough, diphtheria
1960s-onwards	sexually transmitted diseases
1970s-onwards	AIDS epidemic worldwide and transfusion-associated viruses
1980s-onwards	several antibiotic resistant bacteria (e.g., methicillin-resistant *Staphylococcus aureus*, vancomycin-resistant *Enterococcus faecalis*, penicillin-resistant *Streptococcus pneumoniae*, multiresistant enteric bacteria) international foodborne illnesses
New millennium	threats of biohazards and bioterrorism SARS (Severe Acute Respiratory Syndrome) new influenza pandemics

Food for Thought

1. Describe incidents from your own personal experience as a health care professional which attest to the relevance of infection control in everyday practice.
2. Describe incidents from your own personal experience as a lay member of society which attest to the relevance of infection control in everyday practice.
3. What was Pasteur's 'germ theory', and how was its validity challenged in subsequent decades?
4. Distinguish between colonization and infection.
5. What current preventative interventions for infection have contributed to improved newborn health and child health?
6. Why would it be anticipated that infectious diseases would have major impact on the outcome of war or famine?

Supplemental Reading

Azzone GF. *Medicine From Art to Science: The Role of Complexity and Evolution.* Amsterdam:IOS Press, 1998.
- very complex and advanced reading for the critical thinking enthusiast

Cartwright FF, Biddiss M. *Disease and History.* Surrey, UK:Sutton Publishing Ltd., 2004.
- a compilation of epidemics throughout history

Conrad LI, Wujastyk D. *Concepts of Contagion: Perspectives From Pre-Modern Societies.* London, UK:Kegan Paul Intl., 2005.
- a discussion of contagion in China, India, Middle East, and Europe

Gregg CT. *A Virus of Love and Other Tales of Medical Detection.* Albuquerque, USA:University of New Mexico Press, 1985.
- a fiction of science; good fun!

Oldstone MBA. *Viruses, Plagues, and History.* New York:Oxford University Press, 2009.
- a practical concise exposé

Prinzing F. *Epidemics Resulting From Wars.* London:Oxford Press, 1916.
- an old but interesting text

"I study the lives on a leaf; the little
Sleepers, numb nudgers in cold dimensions,
Beetles in caves, newts, stone-deaf fishes,
Lice tethered to long limp subterranean weeds,
Squirmers in bogs,
And bacterial creepers."

William Roethke
The Minimal, 1948

II. It's a Microbe's World !

Organizing the Body of Knowledge

Causes of infection as we generally know them are described as **microbes** on a generic basis. Microbes include a large number of species that are most often very difficult to see with the naked eye. Historically, it was recognized that individual microbes could only be visualized by some form of microscopy; the tiny size led to the derivation of the word microbe. Whereas the word **germ** could be used to describe any microbe which is capable of causing a change in food, human health environment, among other things, germ is more commonly used to describe a microbe that is capable of causing human infection. If microbes are the cause of infections, then we can only appreciate infection control if we have insight into the microbial world.

There are very complex scientific ways to classify microbes into more specific groupings. It is of value to recognize these specific groupings from a scientist's or physician's view because common or specific patterns of infection can be realized as can the common or specific ways to diagnose, treat, and prevent infection. The term **taxonomy** refers to the scientist's approach to formally categorize microbes into related and individual groupings. A review of high school biology notes will no doubt quickly remind us of the strata of classifications that are used to categorize plants, animals, and microbes. The stratified and detailed ascension from phylum to subspecies is of some interest to us but yet of more immediate concern to the biology student who faces the prospect of an examination. From general categorization to very specific

Table 1. Examples of family, genus, species name of medically important bacteria.

Family	Enterobacteriaceae	Pseudomonadaceae	Vibrionaceae
Genus	Escherichia	Pseudomonas	Vibrio
Species	coli	aeruginosa	cholerae

grouping, the hierarchy of descriptive terms includes: Phylum, Subphylum, Class, Order, Family, Genus, Species, and Subspecies. Each microbe can be described by its association with others in each of these categories and then ultimately to its specific name (Table 1). On a practical basis, however, much more simple approaches are used to convey the relationship of microbes to one another.

Whereas it may be of value to understand the relationship of microbes to each other, and whereas it is critical to understand the important features of individual germs, a practical categorization of microbes can be achieved by simply considering that they may be one of four major groups: **viruses**, **bacteria**, **fungi**, and **parasites** (Table 2). There is an apparent exception to these four groups called **prions**. It is much easier to generally categorize germs in the latter format than remember the former scientific biological classifications.

If we look at size alone, there are significant differences among the four broad groups (Table 3). Viruses are the smallest of germs whereas parasites are the largest; bacteria and fungi are typically intermediate although some forms of medically important fungi may be as large as some small parasites. If we look at complexity of design and function, again viruses are most simple, then followed by bacteria, fungi, and parasites respectively in increasing order of complexity. Both viruses and bacteria are designated as **procaryotes** because of their simple design and structure. They carry their own genetic material (DNA or RNA or both) which promotes replication and function, and they have simple organizations of essential machinery within a limiting barrier (i.e., cell membrane). Fungi and parasites are generally more complex. The latter have more complex DNA and cellular functions. Their DNA will be organized into a nucleus where critical replicative and signal functions occur, while much of the day-to-day work of processing nutrients or producing non-DNA building blocks (e.g., proteins) will occur in their cytoplasm which is exterior to the nucleus but still within the membrane boundary which defines their structure.

Table 2. Examples of medically-important microbes in each broad microbial group.

Virus	Bacterium
Herpes simplex	*Escherichia coli*
Polio virus	*Staphylococcus aureus*
Rubella virus	*Neisseria meningitidis*
Measles virus	*Streptococcus pyogenes*
Influenza virus	*Haemophilus influenzae*

Fungus	Parasite
Candida albicans	*Giardia duodenalis*
Cryptococcus neoformans	*Cryptosporidium*
Aspergillus fumigatus	*Entamoaeba histolytica*
Coccidioides immitis	*Taenia solium*
Histoplasma capsulatum	*Schistosoma mansoni*

Table 3. Comparative sizing of the microbial world [*note*: a human red blood cell is approximately 6-8 microns (μm.)].

	Actual size	Comparative sizes
Tapeworm (large parasite)	1metre	100 kilometres
Protozoan (small parasite, e.g., *Cryptosporidium*) or Yeast (an example of a fungus, e.g., *Candida albicans*)	10-100 μm.	1 metre ($\sim 10^{-5}$ smaller than the above)
Gram positive coccus (bacterium, e.g., *Streptococcus pyogenes*)	1-2 μm.	10 cm. (10^{-1} smaller than the above; 10^{-6} smaller than the above tapeworm)
Smallpox virus	0.3 μm.	$\sim$1 cm. (10^{-1} smaller than the above; 10^{-7} smaller than the above tapeworm)
Enterovirus	0.03 μm.	$\sim$1 mm. (10^{-1} smaller than the above; 10^{-8} smaller than the above tapeworm)

In each of the four broad categories, we can define further broad groups which are more narrowly related, and then ultimately even further define particular **species**. Even within a species, however, there are descriptions of related or unrelated groups. All of us have encountered the name *E. coli* which is the common use abbreviation for the species *Escherichia coli*. The two words are a name which include a generic bacterial grouping, hence **genus**, (*Escherichia*) while the "*coli*" provides the species designation. There are other species of the *Escherichia* genus, each with their own particular name (e.g., *Escherichia hermanii* = *E. hermanii*) (Figure 1). *E. coli* can normally be isolated from a majority of humans, specifically as part of usual bowel contents. If we were to attempt to grow *E. coli* in the laboratory from a series of individuals, each individual laboratory isolation of *E. coli* would be called an **isolate**. These isolates are all examples of *E. coli*, but they may or may not vary for other than species-defining characteristics. Most *E. coli* isolates are relatively similar and not of harm in the human gastrointestinal tract. Their presence is actually essential to normal bowel function. There are exceptions, however, and other *E. coli* may possess traits which lead them to be "pathogenic" (i.e., causes of infection). Some *E. coli* may have the ability to produce unique toxins or to attach specially, making them more able to cause diarrhea or urinary tract infections respectively. The pathogenic *E. coli* are no less *E. coli* species, but now have variation in other parts of their genetic make-up (outside of the stable areas of their chromosome that confers their species designation) which makes them disease causing or unique from other *E. coli*. When we are able to show uniqueness among a series of *E. coli* isolates, we call these **strains** of the species. If in an outbreak of toxigenic *E. coli*-related diarrhea which may have been acquired from a common food source (e.g., the local meat-cutter's hamburger),

Figure 1. Diversity in the genus *Escherichia* that is found among human isolates.

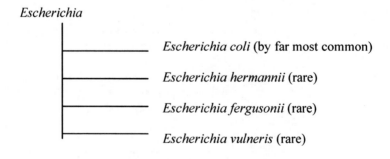

Escherichia

Escherichia coli (by far most common)

Escherichia hermannii (rare)

Escherichia fergusonii (rare)

Escherichia vulneris (rare)

we recognize that 30 people have been infected with a common *E. coli*, we say that a strain of *E. coli* has caused infection. This "strain" designation implies a common source or considerable homology (see Chapter XV). On the other hand, a similar but not absolutely identical toxigenic *E. coli* may be causing diarrhea among patients who are scattered throughout the world whereby there is absolutely no link as far as acquisition is concerned. Despite the common mode for how disease may be produced from any such toxigenic bacterium, these individual **isolates** will be called unique strains. These generalizations of isolate and strain will be relevant to all species whether of viral, bacterial, fungal, or parasite groups.

How do we classify microbes into different groups? Ultimately, genetic techniques allow us to be absolutely precise, but on a more practical basis and with the influence of historical methods, germs can be defined and classified by a number of simple and then modestly complex tests - these are the basis for the work of the diagnostic microbiology laboratory. On an initial basis, microbes, especially bacteria, can be defined by their appearance, either by microscopy (Figures 2 and 3) or macroscopically (unaided eye) after they have been grown by culture techniques in the laboratory. Special staining techniques on the microscope slide may be used to make differences more obvious. Not all germs will actively grow in the laboratory and so some form of microscopy may be the only defining technique. For those microbes where the germ can be cultivated sufficiently in the laboratory, a number of other defining characteristics can be assessed. These may include conditions of growth (atmosphere, time to grow, need for essential nutrients, growth inside and outside of mammalian cells, etc.), phenotypic differences (biochemical/enzyme reactions, toxin presence, antigenic differences, etc.), and genetic differences (i.e., determining the genetic code of various microbes' DNA or RNA sequences). Each species has its unique set of these features. The application of any one technique may be relevant to a group of organisms, but in general, techniques which separate the broad groups are often quite different. Likewise, a group of bacteria may be defined by common techniques, whereas the identification of some exceptional bacteria may require entirely unique methods. Due to this variation, we require consideration of each of the broad groups of viruses, bacteria, fungi, and parasites.

The Virus

Previous to the recognition of **prions** [agents of "mad cow disease": bovine spongiform encephalopathy (BSE)], it had been generally accepted that viruses were the smallest possible infectious particle. Generalizing, viruses are approximately 10-100 times smaller than bacteria and approximately 10-100

Figure 2. Microscopic appearance of bacillus-shaped bacteria by resolution of a typical light microscope. Normally these bacteria would be stained prior to visualizing, and in this particular example, the stain would colour the bacteria purple. The magnification is approximately 1000 times.

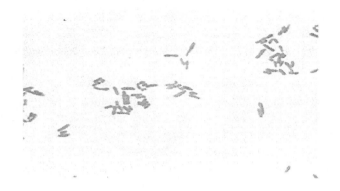

Figure 3. Microscopic appearance of an adenovirus as seen by electron microscopy. Electron microscopy magnifies more than the light microscope but is usually used only for viruses. The magnification is approximately 500,000 times.

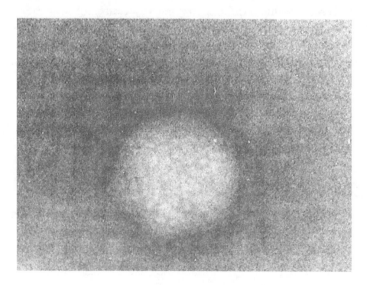

million times smaller than a six foot tall person. Viruses are so small that they cannot be seen with the routine light microscope.

There are many groups of viruses, each having a specific structural and genetic make-up (Figure 4). In general, a virus will have either DNA or RNA as its main genetic constituent. The genetic material will be contained within a solid structural membrane. Some viruses will have an external envelope which surrounds the virus proper. This envelope is of importance to the control of some viruses because it makes them more susceptible to disinfectants. A good example of a virus that lacks this membrane and that is generally resistant in environmental conditions is the poliovirus (a form of enterovirus). This fact allows us to realize how such a virus could be transmitted to a susceptible individual via potable water supplies. For some viruses, the genetic material is segmented (i.e., not a single length of DNA or RNA, but rather many separate lengths). It is believed that such structure facilitates the development of mutant viruses due to the potential for their genetic material to more easily re-assort. This ability to re-assort for some viruses, along with any virus' ability to have its genetic material mutate, will lead to strain variation or escape mutants. For example, influenza pandemics are believed to occur when the virus RNA changes lead to major alterations in virus surface proteins that are recognized by the body's immune system (Figure 5). The immune system cannot recognize the newly changed virus and thus must relearn to develop protection. In another example, the human immunodeficiency ("AIDS") virus is able to easily generate mutants when exposed to antiviral agents. For the latter virus, such resistant mutants are developed almost as fast as new pharmaceuticals are developed and implemented. The potential variation of genetic material for a given virus will mean that many different variants of the same virus can exist (e.g., enteroviruses are numbered as over 70 different types; e.g., adenoviruses are numbers to over 40 different types). These differences will often mean that the body must mount a large spectrum of immune responses in order to be resistant to all of the given virus' variants (i.e., infection due to one enterovirus will not always allow the body to develop resistance to the next strain of enterovirus). This will explain why humans may be infected at different times with many different cold viruses (rhinoviruses).

Viruses are replication cripples: their machinery and genetic content are so simple, relatively speaking, that they do not have the ability to reproduce by themselves (Figure 6). Unlike the majority of bacteria, parasites, and fungi, viruses require entry into the human cell in order to be reproduced. The virus will at first attach itself to the cell of first encounter. The human cell will facilitate the infection by internalizing the virus. Once inside the cell, the virus' genetic material, either DNA or RNA, will be reproduced by the human cell machinery

Figure 4. Schematic representations of different virus structures. The circular structures around the rhinovirus and retrovirus represent viral 'coats'.

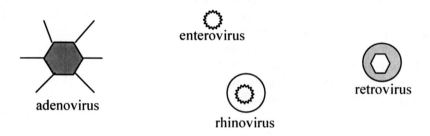

enterovirus

adenovirus

rhinovirus

retrovirus

Figure 5. Schematic drawing of influenza virus. The interior of the virus has eight separate elements of genetic material (RNA). The surface of the virus has both hemagglutinin (black) and neuraminidase (grey) structures which facilitate binding of the virus but which are quite susceptible to structural shifts as a consequence of the potential for genetic alterations when the genetic material changes.

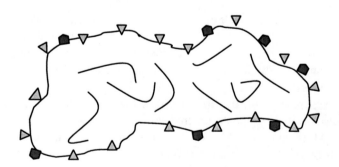

Figure 6. Life cycle of a human herpesvirus. The virus is normally coated with a fatty envelope which fuses with the human cell border. In the cytoplasm, the virus is uncoated of this envelope and begins to instigate the formation of early virus proteins. The formation of the main structure of the virus and the packaging of replicated DNA occur in the nucleus. As the newly formed virus escapes the nucleus, it again acquires an envelope and then exits the human cell.

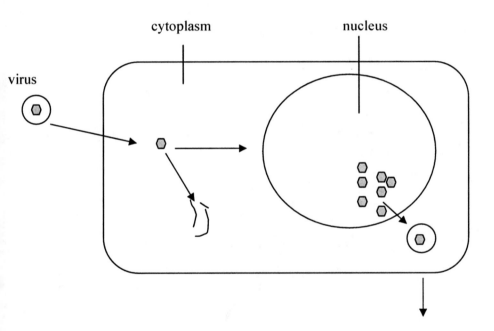

under the virus' influence. Other components of the virus will be assembled, and an entire virus is then free in the human cell's cytoplasm. Whereas some viruses will escape the cell and leave it relatively unharmed, others will replicate to the point where the cell may burst or otherwise die. Furthermore, particular viruses may have a predilection for infecting only certain types of human cells in contrast to others which are able to cause widespread disease throughout the body (e.g., hepatitis B virus replicates mainly in liver cells; e.g., enterovirus can infect almost any cell type). Given all of the potential variations relating to structure, genetic content, and cell tropism that we have detailed, it is not surprising to realize that virus infections are quite varied in their clinical manifestations. On a practical basis, these features of virus replication necessitate that they be detected from clinical samples by growth in laboratory mammalian cell lines - it requires several days to weeks to isolate and characterize a virus.

Table 4 outlines some key features of important and representative virus groups and as well, an outline of their associated infections. As a group, viruses cause a majority of all infections worldwide. The ways in which they are spread are variable. There are few viruses for which we have antiviral antibiotics to treat, and this limitation remains a major problem in dealing with the infections that they cause.

Table 4. Major viral groups, attributes, and associated common illnesses.

Viruses that have a DNA genome

virus family	virus	attributes	associated illnesses
Adenoviridae			
	adenovirus	non-enveloped, medium sized	upper and lower respiratory, gastroenteritis
Hepadnaviridae			
	hepatitis B	DNA covered with 'surface antigen'	hepatitis, liver cancer
Herpesviridae			
	herpes simplex	enveloped, larger (than above) virus	genital, lip, and skin lesions, rare systemic complications
	herpes zoster	enveloped, larger virus	chicken pox, zoster eruptions
	cytomegalovirus	enveloped, larger virus	congenital infection, generalized infections, infections of compromised patients
	Epstein-Barr virus	enveloped, larger virus	mononucleosis
	human herpes-virus 6 and 7	enveloped, larger virus	roseola, generalized infections
	human herpes-virus 8	enveloped, larger virus	Kaposi's sarcoma
Papoviridae			
	papilloma virus	nonenveloped, small virus	warts, some contribute to female cervical cancer
	polyoma virus	nonenveloped, small virus	central nervous system and urinary tract illnesses among immune compromised patients

Table 4. Cont'd.

Parvoviridae

| | parvovirus (including bocavirus) | nonenveloped, small virus | Fifth's disease (congenital infection, hemolytic anemia); respiratory and GI infections |

Poxviridae

	smallpox	very large, enveloped virus	smallpox (vaccinia is the vaccine version)
	molluscum contagiosum virus	very large, enveloped virus	vesicular skin rash
	Orf virus	very large, enveloped virus	skin lesion (a zoonosis)

Viruses that have a RNA genome

virus family	virus	attributes	associated illnesses
Arenaviridae			
	Lassa fever virus	enveloped, segmented genome, small virus	Lassa fever (systemic illness; geographically restricted)
	lymphocytic choriomeningitis virus	enveloped, segmented genome, small virus	central nervous system infection (a zoonosis)
Bunyaviridae			
	California encephalitis virus	enveloped, segmented genome, small virus	systemic illness including central nervous system (arthropod transmitted and several variants)
	LaCrosse virus	enveloped, segmented genome, small virus	systemic illness including central nervous system
Caliciviridae			
	Norwalk-like	nonenveloped, small virus	gastroenteritis
Coronaviridae			
	coronavirus (includes SARS)	enveloped, medium-sized virus	upper and lower respiratory infections

Table 4. Cont'd.

Delta

Delta agent	enveloped, medium-sized	hepatitis co-factor

Filoviridae

Ebola virus	enveloped, small virus	systemic illness (geographically restricted)
Marburg virus	enveloped, small virus	systemic illness (geographically restricted)

Flaviviridae

yellow fever virus	enveloped, small virus	hepatitis, systemic illness (arthropod transmitted)
dengue fever virus	enveloped, small virus	systemic illness, rash (arthropod transmitted)
Japanese encephalitis virus	enveloped, small virus	systemic illness including central nervous system (arthropod transmitted)
St.Louis encephalitis virus	enveloped, small virus	systemic illness including central nervous system (arthropod transmitted)
West Nile-like virus	enveloped, small virus	systemic illness including central nervous system (arthropod transmitted)
tick-borne encephalitis virus	enveloped, small virus	systemic illness including central nervous system (arthropod transmitted)
hepatitis C	enveloped, small virus	hepatitis, liver cancer

Orthomyxoviridae

influenza A, B, and C	enveloped, small virus with multi-segmented genome	upper and lower respiratory disease, systemic illness

Paramyxoviridae

parainfluenza virus	enveloped, small virus	upper and lower respiratory disease
mumps virus	enveloped, small virus	upper respiratory infection, systemic infection including meningitis

Table 4. Cont'd.

metapneumovirus	enveloped, small virus	respiratory infections
measles virus	enveloped, small virus	rash, systemic infection, respiratory infection
respiratory syncytial virus	enveloped, small virus	upper and lower respiratory disease

Picornaviridae

enterovirus (including poliovirus, echo-virus, and coxsackie virus)	nonenveloped, small virus	systemic illness, rashes, heart infection, central nervous system infections
rhinovirus	enveloped, small virus	upper and lower respiratory infections
hepatitis A virus	(like enterovirus)	hepatitis

Reoviridae

rotavirus	non-enveloped, small virus	gastroenteritis
Colorado tick fever virus	non-enveloped, small virus	systemic illness including central nervous system disease (arthropod transmitted and geographically restricted)

Retroviridae

HIV (human immuno-deficiency virus)	enveloped, small virus with segmented genome	immunodeficiency and systemic illness
HTLV I and II	enveloped, small viruses with segmented genomes	systemic infection, central nervous system infection, lymphoid cancer

Rhabdoviridae

rabies virus	enveloped, small virus	rabies (a zoonosis)

Togaviridae

rubella virus	enveloped, small virus	rash, systemic illness
Western equine encephalitis virus	enveloped, small virus	systemic illness including central nervous system illness (arthropod transmitted and geographically restricted)

Table 4. Cont'd.

Eastern equine encephalitis virus	enveloped, small virus	systemic illness including central nervous system illness (arthropod transmitted and geographically restricted)
Venezuelan encephalitis virus	enveloped, small virus	systemic illness including central nervous system illness (arthropod transmitted and geographically restricted)

The Bacterium

Examine a metric ruler and revisit the centimetre. Divide the centimetre by 1000 to 10,000 times and you will approximate the size of most bacteria. Bacteria, therefore, can only be visualized individually by the conventional light microscope. In the laboratory, bacteria are detected when viewed under the microscope either after staining samples of the microbe directly or after staining a microscope slide smear of human specimen with a particular process known as the **Gram stain**. Apart from actually staining the bacteria, this process will then differentiate among bacteria as we will later discuss.

In general, bacteria divide by the process of **binary fission** (i.e., a single bacterium elongates and then divides into two) (Figure 7). In the laboratory, fairly simple culture conditions, such as a soybean digest fluid or a meat broth, will allow growth for most bacteria. Whereas the conditions of bacterial growth can be regulated in the laboratory, circumstances are much different in the human where a number of factors either facilitate or inhibit growth. For common bacteria, such as *Escherichia coli* (generally known as *E. coli*), laboratory conditions can provide for bacterial doubling times as short as 30 minutes. When one extrapolates the exponential doubling time over a twenty-four hour period, it is not surprising to realize that large "**colonies**" of bacteria will be obtained in short order (Figure 8). Therefore, the *E. coli* cause of a urinary tract infection may be realized as such at least one to two days after the acquisition of the patient's urine. Whereas most bacteria will grow easily and rapidly, others may have doubling generation times which range from hours to days (e.g., the bacterial cause of tuberculosis, *Mycobacterium tuberculosis*, may require two to six weeks in order to be cultured and hence recognized in the laboratory).

Figure 7. Diagramatic representation of binary fission as the mode of replication for bacteria. Stepwise progression of enlargement, septation, elongation, and division occur endlessly in a cyclical fashion.

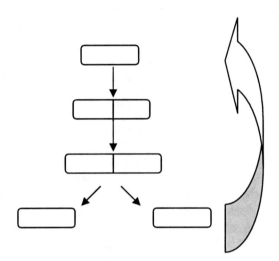

Figure 8. Photograph of bacterial colonies growing on an agar medium.

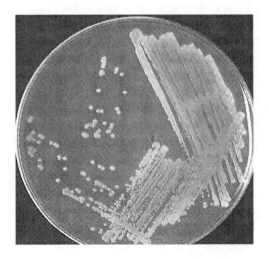

Rarely, some unusual bacteria will not grow in artificial laboratory media and may require conditions very similar to viruses. Still others are not grown outside of laboratory animals which have been infected, and therefore a culture diagnosis of the infection may not be practical (e.g., the cause of syphilis, *Treponema pallidum*, cannot be grown with conventional laboratory culture techniques).

Bacteria which grow in the laboratory from clinical specimens will require a mixture of nutrients. These may include amino acids, carbohydrates, vitamins, lipids, minerals, and water. A large variety of such growth media are possible. Whereas these growth media can be liquid, they can also be solidified by the addition of agar (a seaweed extract) which functions to harden the medium comparable to the effects of pectin in a jam or jelly. The value of these solid media is that actual colonies of bacteria can be grown and visualized. In this form, the laboratory may then perform a number of investigations which will classify the particular germ. Some human pathogens require more complete growth substrates, and these may include animal blood components. In addition to growth substrates, growth temperature and atmosphere may be very important. In general, human pathogenic bacteria grow well at 35-37°C. **Aerobic** bacteria will grow under conditions of usual atmospheric gas whereas others (**anaerobes**) will grow only in an atmosphere where the oxygen content is depleted. Still others (**capnophiles**) will require carbon dioxide or slight reduction in ambient oxygen (**microaerophilic**). Many common bacteria (e.g., streptococci, staphylococci, and *E. coli*) can grow in any atmosphere or body condition. When we look at all of the factors that may be required for the growth and sustenance of the large spectrum of simple or fastidious bacteria, the body is able to provide many if not all of these requirements, and as it is, the human body can be infected with a great diversity of bacteria.

The structure of bacteria is critical to the understanding of how they behave during infections (Figure 9). The bacterial cytoplasm, where genetic material and machinery exists, is contained by a cell membrane. External to this membrane, most bacteria have a cell wall which varies in complexity and constituents depending on the species. The cell wall and membrane complex are critical sites where, for example, the Gram stain dyes bind differentially to some bacteria and not others. This complex also maintains structures which are the sites of action for penicillin and similar antibiotics. To make things even more complex, some bacteria have capsular structures external to the cell wall; the latter can resist the attack of the body's white blood cells. Some of these capsules when purified, however, may serve as vaccines. **Flagella** are whip-like proteins that facilitate motility (Figure 10). Other hair-like projections called **pili** or **fimbriae** serve as communication lines to similar bacteria or attachment cables to human cells. A few bacteria (e.g., *Bacillus* species, *Clostridium* species)

Figure 9. Schematic representation of a general bacterial cell.

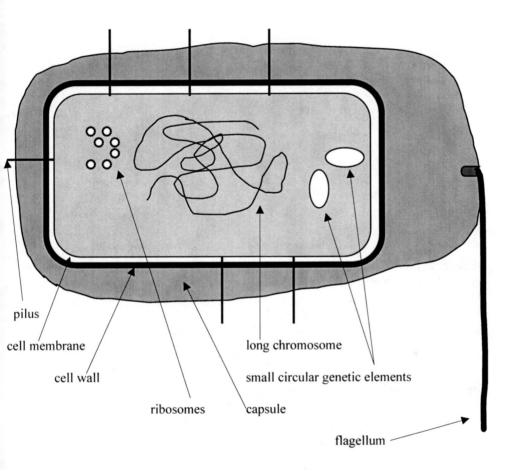

pilus

cell membrane

cell wall

ribosomes

long chromosome

small circular genetic elements

capsule

flagellum

are capable of producing sessile, dormant forms called **spores** (Figure 11). These spores are relatively heat resistant and allow for survival in extreme environmental conditions. When circumstances are right, the spores will transform back into active replicating bacteria analogous to a seed that grows into

34

Figure 10. Electronmicroscopic appearance of a bacterium with multiple flagella. This example is that of *Treponema* which is linked to the illness called syphilis. The bacterium has been magnified some 50,000 times.

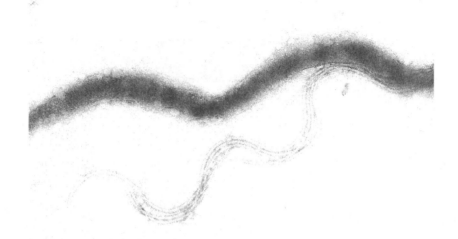

Figure 11. Electronmicroscopic appearance of a bacterium with an internal spore. This example is that of *Bacillus cereus* which can cause food poisoning. The bacterium has been magnified some 45,000 times.

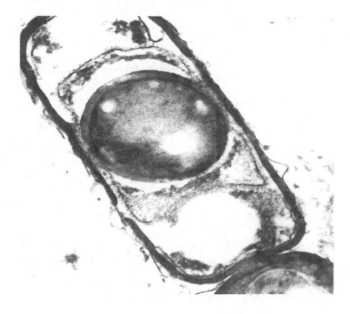

a viable plant. Most important is that spore-forming organisms are capable of withstanding heat and therefore may serve as potential causes of food poisoning when heat-prepared foods allow for spore germination at a later time (Table 5).

The main bacterial genetic code material is DNA, usually in the form of a long chromosome. Additionally, some bacteria have additional bits of DNA called plasmids. Essential genes are maintained on the chromosome while these additional DNA fragments maybe responsible for the production of various enzymes, antibiotic resistant traits, or **virulence factors** (factors which promote the disease potential of the bacterium). Whereas bacteria have a number of inherent characteristics which allow for infection or seclusion from the human defence system, bacteria are also able to cope with change and stress by mutation. Parts of the DNA continually mutate and, if the bacteria are exposed to some form of selective pressure, some of the natural mutants will have spontaneously changed to a state where they have developed a new coping mechanism. In addition, some bacteria can exchange genetic material between members of their own species or, more uncommonly, between themselves and members of other bacterial species. Bacteria also have the ability to take up DNA from the environment, again possibly incorporating this DNA in their own structures to allow for subsequent genetic change. Overall, it is obvious that bacteria may change in order to meet the demands of life.

Once grown in the laboratory, bacteria can be identified by various techniques (Tables 6, 7, and 8). For example, they may be initially classified by their staining pattern (Gram stain reaction), appearance of bacterial colonies, and atmosphere of growth. Furthermore, biochemical analyses may determine the ability of bacteria to utilize certain growth substrates or produce a variety of enzymes. A complex profile of these abilities will then determine the species (i.e., the pattern is almost like a fingerprint for determining the identification). Likewise, identification can be facilitated by analyses of the types of cell wall or capsule constituents with the use of immunological tests. The

Table 5. Examples of spore-forming bacteria that cause food poisoning.

bacterium	source	contamination	illness	food commonly affected
Bacillus cereus	environmental (e.g., dust, soil)	direct contact, airborne	emesis, diarrhea	pre-cooked rice
Clostridium perfringens	mammalian intestinal	direct contact	diarrhea	meat products

Table 6. Methods that are used to classify bacteria in a diagnostic laboratory.

I.   Appearance/morphology of colonies after laboratory culture.

II.   Staining reactions (e.g., Gram stain; e.g., Ziehl-Neelsen stain).

III.   Atmospheric/oxygen growth requirements.

IV.   Biochemical tests (e.g., tests of metabolism, growth requirements, etc.)

V.   Serological tests (assessment of structure by immune reactions).

VI.   Genetic determinations (i.e., unique sequence of DNA or RNA may be specific for microbial determination).

Table 7. Components of the Gram stain – one of the most commonly used diagnostic tests in the study of routine bacteria from clinical samples or bacterial cultures.

A.   Microscopic glass slide is smeared with clinical sample or bacterium. The smear is gently heat-fixed or air-dried.

B.   The slide is overlaid with a solution of crystal violet (purple).

C.   After washing the above with water, the slide is overlaid with a solution of 'Gram's iodine'. Gram positive bacteria have a cellular constituent which will allow the iodine component to fix the crystal violet firmly onto the bacterium.

D.   After washing the above with water, the slide is exposed to a specific alcohol wash which removes the crystal violet and iodine from bacteria that do not possess the Gram positive binding component.

E.   A safranin or fuchsin solution is overlaid onto the slide and then washed off with water after a particular incubation period.

F.   Gram positive bacteria have retained the iodine-crystal violet complex and thus appear purple.

Gram negative bacteria have had the iodine-crystal violet complex washed off by the alcohol solution but are nevertheless stained by the safranin or fuchsin solution, and thus appear red. Some rare bacteria will not stain at all by either approach and yet others stain incompletely (these are call Gram variable).

Table 8. Examples of laboratory tests which are used for bacterial identification and which may be spoken of in the context of clinical infections and infection control.

Coagulase test – a determination of the ability of a bacterium to coagulate a specific animal serum. The test differentiates staphylococci. 'Coagulase-positive' staphylococci are synonymous with *Staphylococcus aureus* – the most pathogenic staphylococcus. 'Coagulase-negative' staphylococci are much less virulent and often are contaminants.

Hemolysis – the ability of bacteria to break down red blood cells is determined. When screening throat swab cultures for *Streptococcus pyogenes* ('strep throat'), one looks for 'hemolytic' bacterial colonies on a culture medium that contains whole red blood cells.

Lactose fermentation – ability of a bacterium to ferment the carbohydrate lactose. This is a key reaction in the differentiation of diarrheal pathogens such *Salmonella* and *Shigella* species from non-pathogenic Gram negative bacilli that are found normally in the intestines.

Carbohydrate fermentation or utilization – as for lactose fermentation, a determination is made of the ability of a bacterium to ferment or make use of a series of carbohydrates. The negative or positive reactions are turned into a binary or similar numeric code which will identify a bacterium.

Oxidase test – a colourimetric reaction which determines the ability of a bacterium to possess a specific metabolic/energy pathway. When applied to Gram negative rods and found positive, the test broadly categorizes them into some bacteria that resemble *Pseudomonas* species in contrast to others.

schemata which are used to stratify bacteria for identification are quite complex. Figures 12 a, b, and c outline such schemata for medically important germs.

Not all bacteria of a given species are capable of producing disease. Some are more capable than others because they possess special abilities to produce toxins or attachment factors. Variations in their structures, such as presence of capsules, will also confer different disease-causing potential. Some will be capable of producing enzymes that are able to modify antibiotics, hence inactivating these antibiotics.

Bacterial species are numerous throughout nature and only a limited number are capable of causing human disease (see XIX. Profile of Medically Relevant Bacteria). Bacteria are also capable of being very beneficial and in general these beneficial bacteria do not cause infection (e.g., yoghurt-fermenting bacteria or vinegar-producing bacteria).

38

Figure 12a. The crash course in bacterial taxonomy.

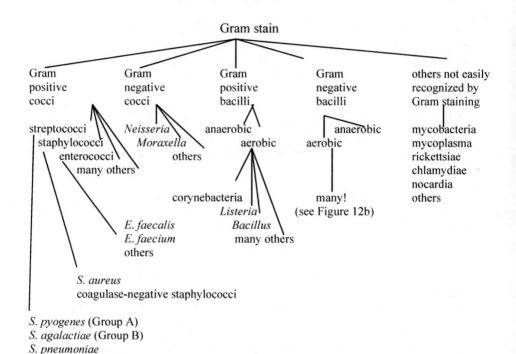

Figure 12b. Further strata of aerobic Gram negative bacilli.

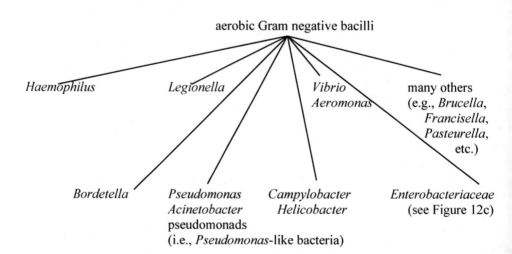

Figure 12c. Further strata of the bacterial family called *Enterobacteriaceae*.

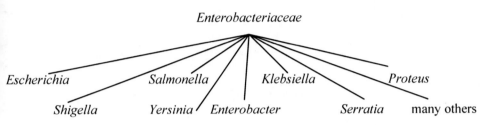

The Fungus

Most of us will recognize the word **fungus**, but reserve our memory to rekindle visions of some form of delectable mushroom which may grace our hors d'oeuvres or primi piatti. The population of fungi in nature is considerably diverse, and among these only a limited number (by far, the vast minority) may actually cause human infection or other diseases. Again, some of these organisms may be of benefit (e.g., cooking, cheese ripening, antibiotic production, brewing).

Disease causing fungi generally take few forms (see Figures 13 a and b). Some are shaped as round or oval forms called **yeast**. Yeast are slightly larger than bacteria. Other fungi may be filamentous and are called **molds**. Molds produce tubular structures referred to as **hyphae** which may or may not bear environment-resistance spores. The latter spores are not as heat or chemical resistant as bacterial spores. Mold hyphae are long enough to be visible to the naked eye (e.g., the fuzzy parts of fruit mold). A few other fungi of medical concern are capable of existing in either the yeast or mold form depending on the laboratory conditions (Table 9).

Fungi are much more complex than viruses or bacteria. The structure of their genetic material is more similar to human cells or parasites. As a result, their growth, reproduction, and other capabilities are proportionately more complex. Nevertheless, they are capable of being grown on relatively simple media in the laboratory.

Figure 13 a. Photograph of a yeast (*Candida albicans*). These are spherical forms which may have buds. This representation has been captured in a Gram stain which has been magnified some 1000 times under the microscope.

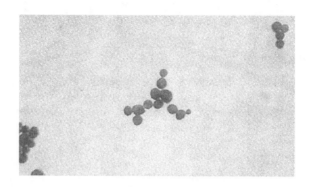

Figure 13b. Photograph of a mold. A mold would grow in the laboratory similar to a fuzzy mold which is seen on fruit. The photograph below captures the appearance as seen under the microscope and magnified some 500 times. Note both the filamentous hyphae and the fungal spores both of which belong to the same mold.

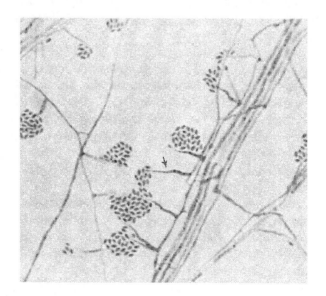

Table 9. Categorization and examples of medically-important fungi.

name	associations
yeast	
Candida albicans	common normal flora, invasive infections in compromised hosts, thrush, vaginitis, diaper rash
other *Candida* species	less common normal flora, invasive infections in compromised hosts
Cryptococcus	environmental source, invasive infections in compromised hosts
several others	
molds	
'dermatophytes'	human, animal, and environmental sources; this group includes several species (e.g., *Microsporum*, *Epidermophyton*, *Trichophyton*) that infect superficial skin and nails
Aspergillus	environmental source, allergic reactions rarely, invasive infections in compromised hosts
Mucor	environmental source, invasive infections in compromised hosts
many others	mainly environmental, are causes of infection

dimorphic fungi (capable of both yeast and mold forms)

name	associations
Histoplasma capsulatum	environmental foci that are geographically restricted, has invasive potential
Coccidiodes immitis	environmental foci that are geographically restricted, has invasive potential
Blastomyces dermatitidis	environmental foci that are geographically restricted, has invasive potential
Paracoccidioides braziliensis	environmental foci that are geographically restricted, has invasive potential
few others	

special

name	associations
Pneumocystis jirovecii (formerly *P. carinii*)	environmental, originally thought to be a parasite, it is believed that the microbe more closely resembles fungi; causes mainly pulmonary disease

Fungi are very common in the environment with the exception of some yeast which may be part of the normal microbes found in different parts of the body in small numbers (e.g., yeast in the oral cavity, bowel, and female genital tract). Fungi are generally unique in the pattern of infections that they cause. In fact, apart from some superficial infections such as those of skin, mouth, and female genital tract, fungi are more likely to infect individuals who have very suppressed immune systems. They are also unique in being susceptible to a very narrow spectrum of antibiotics, often those which have no effect on bacteria (see Chapter IX).

Although we know that some fungi can actively infect humans, there are other forms of disease, not infection, that may be associated with a limited number. Mushroom poisonings, other food poisonings due to overgrowth contamination, and airborne allergies from environmental fungi are examples of these non-infectious diseases.

The Parasite

The term **parasite** is understood in different ways. On a strict scientific basis, the word refers to a specific subset of the microbial world which we discuss herein. In lay or more general terms, parasite is also used to describe a living form which lives off another living form; this is not the connotation which we use in this section. In otherwise describing the interaction of any infecting microbe and the human or other mammal which it infects, we can use 'parasite' to refer to the germ in general terms. Thus, when we describe the host-parasite relationship, we detail the interactions of germ and animal.

The parasites which infect humans are relatively few in numbers compared to the vast array of bacteria. Parasites can be subdivided into several groups which may vary considerably in their structure and mechanism of disease causation. Some parasites are as small as yeasts (protozoa). They may be unicellular or multicellular. Whereas the simple unicellular parasites may be capable of performing several functions as a complete living unit, other more complex parasites are multi-cellular and may have specialized cells which carry out unique functions (e.g., flatworms, roundworms). The latter parasites can be sufficiently large so to be seen by the unaided eye, and indeed many parasites may achieve impressive if not concerning lengths (e.g., some tapeworms can be several metres long). The latter more complex parasites resemble higher orders of life with such specialized tissue. Figure 14 details important parasites of concern for human infection.

Figure 14. Key parasites of medical importance.

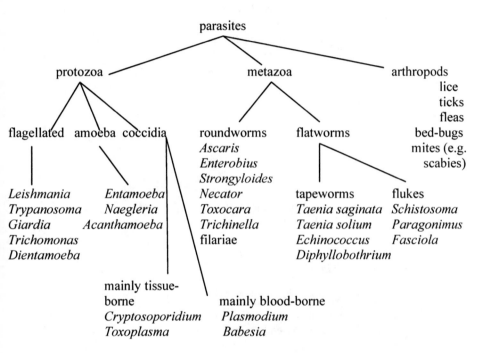

In general, parasites often have complex life cycles (Figure 15). Part of this cycle includes human infection, and the other life cycle components usually include a form of infection or maturation in another living form or in the environment. Each parasite tends to have a rather unique life cycle, and furthermore, parasites will often differ with respect to tropism for particular body tissues (Table 10). Person-to-person spread is important for very few parasites, and transmission from food, insect vector, or environment is often critical.

In addition to parasites that may invade the body or cause gastrointestinal infections, others may cause very superficial skin infections or infestations; these are often referred to as ectoparasites (e.g., scabies, lice, bed bugs, ticks). Some ectoparasites are capable of transmitting viral or bacterial infections (e.g., mosquito for malaria or yellow fever; e.g., ticks for Lyme spirochetes; e.g., body lice for relapsing fever bacteria).

Figure 15. Examples of complex parasite life cycles.

Malaria due to *Plasmodium* species

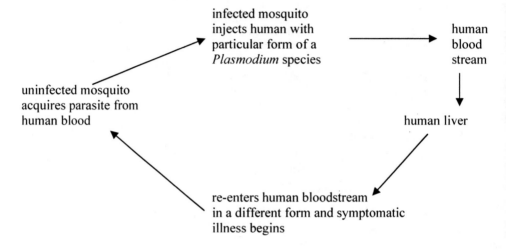

Pinworm (*Enterobius vermicularis*) infection

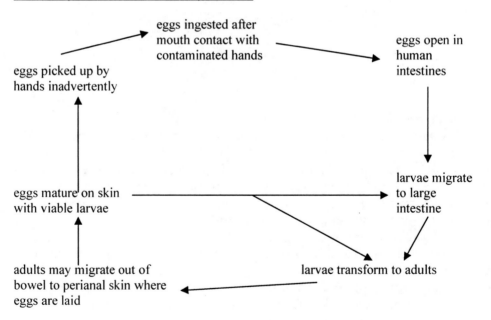

Table 10. Disease associations and source of common human parasites.

parasite	source	main disease association
Protozoa		
Leishmania	sandfly bite	cutaneous or chronic systemic illness
Trypanosoma	fly bite	acute and chronic systemic illnesses depending on specific *Trypanosoma* species
Giardia	human, waterborne	diarrhea
Dientamoeba	unknown	diarrhea, asymptomatic colonization
Trichomonas	human	vaginitis
Entamoeba histolytica	human	diarrhea, rare systemic illness
Naegleria	environmental	rare systemic, topical ocular
Acanthamoeba	environmental	rare systemic, topical ocular
Cryptosporidium	waterborne, animal source	diarrhea
Toxoplasma	feline (e.g. cats)	systemic illnesses
Plasmodium	mosquito	blood-borne (malaria)
Babesia	mosquito	blood-borne
Metazoan		
Ascaris	contaminated food	intestinal mainly (also known as 'roundworm')
Enterobius	humans	perianal (also known as 'pinworm')
Strongyloides	soil	mainly intestinal
Necator	soil	mainly intestinal
Taenia saginata	undercooked beef	mainly intestinal (also known as 'beef tapeworm')
Taenia solium	undercooked pork	intestinal, systemic illness (also known as 'pork tapeworm')
Echinococcus granulosus	eggs ingested accidentally	systemic illness (known as 'hydatid disease')
Diphyllobothrium latum	fish	mainly intestinal (known as 'fish tapeworm')
Schistosoma	environmental sources	systemic (known as 'blood fluke')
Paragonimus	environmental sources	pulmonary (known as 'lung fluke')

Table 10. Cont'd.

Fasciola	environmental sources	hepatic (known as 'liver fluke')
Toxocara	eggs ingested accidentally	systemic infection
Trichinella	uncooked meat	systemic infection, allergic reaction
filariae	mosquitoes, flies	systemic infection

Parasitic infections cause millions of infections worldwide (Table 11), and there are particular geographic distributions depending on climate, presence of vectors, quality of life, food source, among other things. Whereas many parasitic infections will be manifest by particular symptoms and signs, still others may be relatively asymptomatic and persistent. Treatment often requires special anti-parasitic antimicrobials that are inactive against bacterial or fungal causes of infection.

Table 11. Estimated world-wide frequency of some common parasitic infections.

Malaria	~300-500 million active infections per year
Filariasis	>100 million active infections
Chaga's disease (*Trypanosoma cruzi*)	~20 million active infections
Toxoplasma gondii	10-50% of all population have evidence of prior exposure
Giardia	present in ~5% of all stool samples that are submitted for diagnostic parasitology
Cryptosporidium	massive waterborne outbreaks reported throughout the world

To Be Or Not To Be Infectious

Whereas essentially all of the microbes which infect humans are among the aforementioned broad categories, **prions** (from 'protein infectious particles') are currently the single exception to this rule. While having properties of an infectious agent by virtue of the ability to spread from others (animal to human), the prion structure is apparently simplistic. Infection on a practical basis is seemingly only of the central nervous system; in animals, the best example is bovine spongiform encephalopathy ("Mad Cow Disease") and among humans, Creutzfeldt-Jakob Disease (CJD). Central nervous system cells have numerous normal proteins, but one in particular appears to be capable of assuming an unusual structure. When folded in this unusual structure, other similar but normal proteins may become reconfigured into this unusual 'prion' shape by using the abnormal protein as a template, similar to the fine repetitive pattern of a crystal (Figure 16). In essence, the abnormal protein begins a cascade which finalizes in a form of non-senile dementia due to cellular disarray. The abnormal protein will have been inoculated into the human central nervous system by instruments which have been contaminated from another source patient's neurosurgery. The potential for transmission from animal to human through the ingestion of meat has been the focus of much public and medical attention, especially in Europe. Thus, although the protein in itself does not have replicative tools or protective coats or genetic material, it apparently favors the creation of similar harmful proteins and is transmissible. Such concepts are revolutionary.

Figure 16. The prion hypothesis.

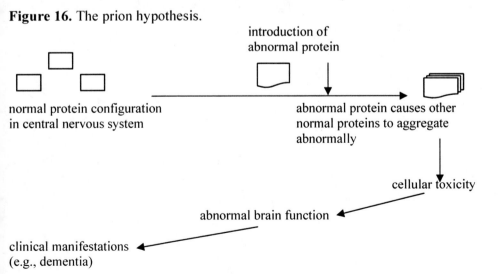

introduction of abnormal protein

normal protein configuration in central nervous system

abnormal protein causes other normal proteins to aggregate abnormally

cellular toxicity

abnormal brain function

clinical manifestations (e.g., dementia)

How They Infect And How They Survive

For any given infection, there will be an interaction between microbe and host which will lead to variation in terms of how the disease will be manifest. On one hand, the disease-causing microbe must have a number of strategies to attach to the host, invade, antagonize, and replicate. On the other hand, the human has natural defence mechanisms which must either be overcome or at least be temporarily side-stepped. The determination of whether there will be an infection, colonization, or simply a passing encounter will depend on the balancing act between the microbe's ability to attack versus the body's ability to defend.

At the initial encounter, the microbe must attach to the site of disease. For pathogens which infect mucous membrane sites (e.g., cold viruses), there is usually an attachment molecule(s) on the host cell (Figure 17). Some pathogens will be inoculated into the body and may avoid the latter need for mucosal contact. Nevertheless, all infecting microbes have a tropism for some specific body tissue. Others may infect all body cells and tissue if given the opportunity

Figure 17. Attachment factor-receptor interaction in bacterial attachment.

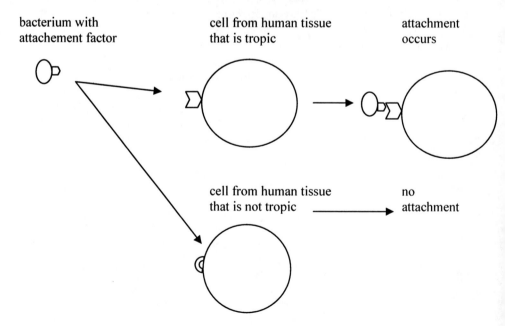

(e.g., some invasive viruses). The need for site-specific attachment is important to recognize because it affords possibilities for disease prevention. For example, if the nasal mucosal site is the entry point for a particular virus, then stimulation of locally protective antibody by vaccination may be of value in protection.

For some microbes, superficial attachment and colonization provide the inaugural step, but the actual disease may be caused by an enzyme or toxin that the microbe thereafter produces. The enzymes may be capable of causing a localized reaction which can subsequently facilitate invasion. The enzymes may destroy cells and tissue. An enzyme may also be one that destroys protective human antibody or one that destroys antibiotics. Some microbes may elaborate toxins that cause a local effect, while other toxins may be carried throughout the body to cause disease at distal sites.

Those microbes which are capable of invading tissue will usually go through replication cycles which continue to cause host cell degeneration. For example, invasive viruses multiply in cells, cause cells to die and burst, and then go on to invade nearby healthy cells in the same pattern. Invasive microbes include examples from all of the four major microbial groups, but viruses are perhaps the best example because they depend on intracellular machinery to reproduce.

Some microbes will not invade cells, and these are termed extracellular pathogens. They are more likely to be recognized at some point in time by host defences. Others that actually invade cells will have an extra measure of protection because the intracellular location in itself serves to hide the pathogens and thus elude host defences. Still others may remain extracellular but will infect host tissue that is relatively secluded. The body's immune response is more likely to have problems defending against an organism which has hidden itself in the central nervous system versus one that is in the blood.

As we shall detail in the next chapter, the body will have numerous host defences, but for each, varied microbes will have evolved ways to counter these protective mechanisms. For example, white blood cells of a certain type engulf and digest some microbes. Yet, unique cell wall components of some bacteria have especially been designed which will resist this "**phagocytosis**".

Microbes are also capable of stimulating a body's response to their favor. While bacteria will consume oxygen in a closed setting (e.g., body cavity), the atmosphere will become right for other bacteria (e.g., anaerobes) to replicate. The inflammatory response to infection as stimulated by a microbe may in itself further propagate the local infection. Inflammation mediators may then cause more tissue damage and swelling.

Microbes may have unique attachment factors, they may be motile, they may have the abilities to produce enzymes which degrade cells, other tissue components, and antibiotics, they may produce toxins which are excreted, they may change their outward appearance ("antigenic coat"), they may have features to resist immunity, and they have complex genetic control and sensory mechanisms which have a feedback loop to facilitate responses to the environment. Whereas some microbes may cause disease on the basis of only one aggressive mechanism (also called **virulence factor**), others may have multiple disease-promoting strengths (Table 12). A good example of these latter is the common bacterium *Staphylococcus aureus* which has attachment factors, invasive enzymes, toxins, antibiotic resistance mechanisms, and antibody degrading and attaching capabilities.

Table 12. Examples of known virulence factors for pathogenic bacteria.

microbe	virulence factor	illness
E. coli O157:H7	verotoxin, attachment factors	diarrhea, systemic illness with kidney failure
Clostridium tetani	tetanus toxin	tetanus
Streptococcus pyogenes	capsule, M protein, proteases, streptolysins, DNAse, exotoxins	strep throat, skin infections, systemic illnesses
Staphylococcus aureus	toxins, coagulase, immunoglobulin binding, tissue lytic enzymes	mainly skin and deep tissue infections
Bordetella pertussis	attachment factors, pertussis toxin	whooping cough
Corynebacterium diphtheriae	diphtheria toxin	diphtheria
Bacillus anthracis	capsule, toxins	anthrax
Yersinia enterocolitica	intracellular multiplication, resistance to immune cells, serum resistance	diarrhea, abdominal pain
Borrelia species	variable outer membrane, motility	Lyme disease, relapsing fever
Neisseria gonorrhoeae	attachment factors, immunoglobulin protease, outer membrane proteins, lipopolysaccharide	gonorrhea, rare systemic infection
Neisseria meningitidis	attachment factors, capsule, immunoglobulin protease, lipopolysaccharide	severe systemic infection, respiratory tract infection, meningitis
Clostridium difficile	enterotoxin, cytotoxin	diarrhea

The ability for microbes to express virulence factors is often a stable part of their genetic makeup. In addition, however, a microbe's capacity to mutate and thus evolve or change is a real threat to the host defence. The latter change is always possible as the ability to mutate is a natural phenomenon of DNA or RNA structure and instability. Supplementary to this ability, though, is the potential for some microbes, especially bacteria, to acquire genetic material from other bacteria, perhaps even from the environment. These recombination events then have the potential to generate newly aggressive or resistant microbes. The survival mechanisms for microbes are in essence no different than the fundamental survival mechanisms for all living forms - faced with adversity, they will most often find a way to cope or change.

A Home Away From Home

The community of microbes that infect us is incredibly diverse. Part of this community takes up permanent residence as normal human microbial flora, and many of these germs are capable of causing infection at some point in time given a facilitative context. Beyond the endogenous microbial flora, however, there is also considerable diversity for where microbes might otherwise survive and thrive.

The simplest of bacteria, for example, can survive in the environment on rudimentary sources of nutrients. Although replication of the microbe may be compromised in a harsh environment, many will persist in a near-dormant stage, only to replicate when the appropriate conditions are met (such as in the human body). Not all of the microbial effects on humans though will require active multiplication in the host. Many microbes are capable of pre-forming harmful toxins (Table 13) or may expose harmful structures after they have multiplied in the environment. Indeed, the actual infection in humans may only be a minor component of the life cycle for many microbes; some will never need a human infection in order to persist in nature.

Soil harbors many bacteria and fungi which can cause infection. Many of the fungi are generally benign but become important when the body's immune system is grossly compromised. *Pseudomonas*-like bacteria are common in soil. *Clostridium tetani* and *Clostridium botulinum*, responsible for tetanus and botulism respectively, are soil microbes.

Water supplies including natural rivers and lakes may have sufficient nutrients for microbial survival. Changes in water temperature and composition may alter the environment to make it more conducive to growth. *Vibrio cholerae*, cause of cholera (a severe form of gastroenteritis), has become a major concern in the Americas due to warm coastal waters. Legionellae, causes of Legionnaire's

Table 13. Examples of human illnesses that are associated with microbial preformed toxins in food.

microbe	toxin	illness
Bacillus cereus	enterotoxins	food poisoning
Clostridium perfringens	enterotoxins	food poisoning
Staphylococcus aureus	enterotoxins	food poisoning
Clostridium botulinum	botulism toxin	acute neurological illness
'ciguatera' fish poisoning (marine microbes)	ciguatera toxin	acute neurological illness
scombroid (multiple bacteria)	histamine	acute histamine response
paralytic shellfish poisoning (marine dinoflagellates)	neurotoxins (e.g., saxitoxin)	acute neurological illness

disease (lower respiratory infections) are present in most sources of fresh water and can be enriched to high quantities if the water is stagnant or if it is warmed to body temperature or slightly higher. Water may become contaminated with fecal organisms from human or other mammals, and these may be carried to us through potable water supplies.

Foods are a major source for human infection. Pathogenic microbes may be present in source meats or vegetables. Meats are not uncommonly tainted with fecal bacteria of animals due to the food harvesting process. The creation of large feed lots and the bulk preparation of food-stuffs have enhanced the ability of infection to be transferred. Vegetables may become tainted with fecal material from natural fertilizer or from contaminated water. Even marine foods may be carriers of pathogenic organisms. Take for example the clam which dwells in an estuary sand and which filters water all day in order to satisfy its own need for organic material. In the process of concentrating these nutrients, it is capable of being a reservoir for diarrhea-causing bacteria, diarrhea-causing viruses, and Hepatitis A virus if these have inadvertently entered the bay water by the dumping of raw sewage in the area. Food-borne illnesses number into the millions if not billions each year; the economic impact from direct patient morbidity is considerable.

Other microbes may be acquired from animals and birds by either direct contact or aerosol. We refer to these as **zoonoses** (Table 14). Individuals who are animal handlers or who work in abattoirs may especially be at risk. Some of

Table 14. Examples of zoonoses and their sources.

	microbe	source	illness
bacteria			
	Borrelia burgdorferi	mammals via specific ticks	Lyme disease
	Brucella species	food	brucellosis (febrile systemic illness)
	Francisella tularensis	mammals either directly or via arthropods	tularemia (febrile systemic illness with localized lymph gland swelling)
	Pasteurella multocida	feline/canine bites	usually localized skin infection
	Yersinia pestis	rodents	plague (different forms)
viruses			
	rabies virus	infected mammals	rabies (neurological illness)
	yellow fever	mosquito	hepatitis, systemic illness
	West Nile-like virus	mosquito	neurological and systemic illness
fungi			
	Microsporum canis	infected pets	skin rash
parasites			
	Echinococcus granulosus	environmental, food	hydatid disease
	Trichinella spiralis	infected undercooked pork	trichinosis

these microbes will cause infections in the source animal as well. The introduction of new animals into an area where they are not endemic is not uncommonly associated with new infection. As an example, *Salmonella* causing diarrhea is usually linked to foods which have been improperly cooked or handled, especially meat-based food of chicken origin. In recent decades, western countries have noted a significant increase in *Salmonella* infection by unusual types which have been imported from other areas of the world via pet turtles, iguanas, other reptiles, and various marsupials and mammals (pigmy hedgehog). Most countries have strict supervision of animal importation.

Human ingenuity has a role to play in newly appearing or re-emerging infections. The creation of new devices and food handling mechanics are a large part of this dilemma. Humidifiers, water tanks, air conditioners, stagnant water pools, among other things have lead to the growth and dissemination of environmental pathogens. The desire to seek the unknown or to explore unhindered nature has created new opportunities to acquire harmful bacteria from animal and the environment.

Just as there are a multitude of harmful microbes, therefore, there are a multitude of foci from which these pathogens may come.

Food for Thought

1. When Gram stains are interpreted for clinical purposes, the clinician integrates microbiological knowledge with clinical knowledge in arriving at a best guess. What most likely bacterium would one be dealing with in the following circumstances?
    a) Gram negative cocci are seen in a sample of cerebrospinal fluid from a patient with meningitis
    b) Gram positive cocci in clusters are seen in a sample of pus which was obtained from a skin abscess
    c) A young female suffers from an active urinary tract infection. Gram negative bacilli are seen in a Gram stain of urine concentrate.
2. Given that a virus will only multiply in the interior of a living human cell, what implications regarding type of infections or forms of immunity might one draw?
3. What beneficial attributes of some fungi have been used for human purposes?
4. With an understanding of the life cycle of the malaria parasite, why do you think that malaria control world-wide has been so problematic?
5. Given the structures of viruses, bacteria, fungi, parasites, and prions, what features do you think would contribute to their susceptibility or resistance to disinfectants?

Supplemental Reading

Cimolai N – ed. *Laboratory Diagnosis of Bacterial Infections*. New York, NY:Marcel Dekker, Inc., 2001.
- advanced reading in bacterial diagnostics with relevant descriptions of basic microbiology and pathogenesis

Greenwood D, Slack R, Peutherer J, Barer M. *Medical Microbiology*. 17th Edition. Philadelphia, USA:Churchill Livingstone Elsevier, 2007.
- a well written and colourful general text with medical emphases

Murray PR, Rosenthal KS, Pfaller MA. *Medical Microbiology*. 6th Edition. Philadelphia, USA:Mosby Elsevier, 2009.
- a well written and colourful general text with medical emphases

Murray PR, Baron EJ, Jorgensen JH, Landry ML, Pfaller MA. *Manual of Clinical Microbiology*. 9th Edition. Washington, DC:ASM Press, 2007.
- an advanced standard in the field of diagnostic microbiology

"Fate gave, what Chance shall not control."
Matthew Arnold
Resignation, 1849

III. The Body's Role

Bacteria On and In the Body Can Be Normal

Privileged areas of the body such as internal organs, muscle and bone, blood, and central nervous system are sterile unless breached by a medical device or procedure. Areas which are exposed either to the environment directly (e.g., skin, external ear, eye) or to a mucosal site (e.g., nose, mouth, gastrointestinal tract, genital tract) inevitably have some bacteria associated with them more or less (Figure 1).

The skin tends to have low numbers of non-pathogenic Gram positive irregular rod-shaped bacteria (often referred to as diphtheroids) and coagulase-negative staphylococci. Occasionally, microbes from the mouth and nose may contaminate skin after having been spread by fingers and saliva. Infants and toddlers may be more prone to the latter, and indeed, usual bowel microbes, like *E. coli*, could contaminate skin in circumstances where good hygiene is not followed, and they may be more commonly present in the diaper region. Further on this theme is concern for the fingernail crypts that may harbor bacteria. Imagine the potential for various bacteria to reside under the fingernail tips of those who change multiple soiled diapers in a toddlers' daycare setting! The external ear and eye surface will also have bacteria which are otherwise seen on the skin, although here again, bacteria may be imported temporarily from nose and mouth by fingers. The end of the urethra in males generally harbors bacteria which are otherwise seen on skin.

Areas that have considerably more and diverse bacteria include the nose, the mouth, the gastrointestinal tract (throughout its entire length), and the female genital tract. Both the nose and mouth have a complex array of Gram positive and Gram negative bacteria. These include organisms which can be aerobic and anaerobic; the latter are more likely to multiply in crypts such as the gingival crevices. Among this diversity, particularly non-pathogenic streptococci ("viridans streptococci" or "mouth streptococci") often predominate.

58

Figure 1. A representation of normal flora of the body.

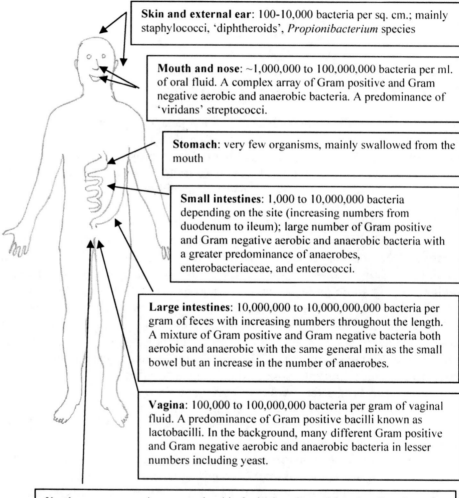

Skin and external ear: 100-10,000 bacteria per sq. cm.; mainly staphylococci, 'diphtheroids', *Propionibacterium* species

Mouth and nose: ~1,000,000 to 100,000,000 bacteria per ml. of oral fluid. A complex array of Gram positive and Gram negative aerobic and anaerobic bacteria. A predominance of 'viridans' streptococci.

Stomach: very few organisms, mainly swallowed from the mouth

Small intestines: 1,000 to 10,000,000 bacteria depending on the site (increasing numbers from duodenum to ileum); large number of Gram positive and Gram negative aerobic and anaerobic bacteria with a greater predominance of anaerobes, enterobacteriaceae, and enterococci.

Large intestines: 10,000,000 to 10,000,000,000 bacteria per gram of feces with increasing numbers throughout the length. A mixture of Gram positive and Gram negative bacteria both aerobic and anaerobic with the same general mix as the small bowel but an increase in the number of anaerobes.

Vagina: 100,000 to 100,000,000 bacteria per gram of vaginal fluid. A predominance of Gram positive bacilli known as lactobacilli. In the background, many different Gram positive and Gram negative aerobic and anaerobic bacteria in lesser numbers including yeast.

Urethra: same organisms as on the skin for both males and females. Females may have contamination from vaginal flora. In children who are diapered, there may be fecal contamination.

Dental caries (cavities) arise when some of the usual oral bacteria degrade the enamel in the presence of food substrate. Whereas much of this microbial burden has very little ability to cause infection, there are small to moderate numbers of various bacteria whose ability to invade the body are much greater. Some of the microbes that are present in low numbers in the mouth include *Staphylococcus aureus*, *Streptococcus pneumoniae*, *Haemophilus influenzae*, *Neisseria meningitidis*, *Streptococcus pyogenes*, and yeast. The reasons for why these latter bacteria remain in check for most individuals will be discussed later. It is not difficult to envision, however, that the illnesses which involve the general area of nose and mouth [e.g., middle ear infection (otitis media), sinus infection (sinusitis)] often include these micro-organisms.

The first major portion of the gastro-intestinal tract is the stomach where the environment is considerably hostile due to extreme acidity which otherwise plays a role in digestion. As saliva is swallowed from the mouth, bacteria from the mouth will follow, but a few of these survive. Thereafter, the numbers of bacteria increase tremendously from the start of the small bowel to the terminal large bowel. In the first portion of the small intestine, there are some coliforms (collection of bacteria resembling and including *E. coli*), enterococci (also known as "fecal streptococci"), various anaerobes, and a few microbes from the mouth which have survived passage through the stomach. The upper small bowel will contain numbers of microbes approaching 10^2-10^5 per ml. Toward the end of the small bowel (terminal ileum), the numbers of bacteria greatly increase to approximately 10^5-10^8 per ml. of intestinal fluid. The bacteria are now predominantly coliforms, enterococci, and anaerobic bacteria. In the large bowel, the numbers reach 10^7-10^9 per ml., and although again the same bacteria predominate, anaerobes often outnumber the rest of the bacteria from ratios of 10:1 to 100:1. Large bowel contents, and therefore faeces, are essentially a mixture of microbes, undigested food, and intestinal mucus and debris. It is not surprising therefore to see that intra-abdominal infections after bowel perforation or major bowel surgery often contain a mixture which reflects the emphasis which is seen in the bowel itself. Odors of intestinal gas and faeces are directly a function of the food we eat which provides growth substances to these bacteria which then yield odorous natural gases (e.g., "H_2S" and particular organic acids). Bacteria in part play a role in breaking down our food, and some are important in nutrient metabolism (e.g., some anaerobes and vitamin K).

The female genital tract also has a complex microbiology, but most microbes will be found in the vagina. Here, there is a great diversity of Gram positive and Gram negative aerobes and anaerobes. Lactobacilli (large Gram positive rods) predominate, and they are able to produce acid by-products from their metabolism; these products will lead to acidification of vagina which in itself mildly decontaminates the site. In small numbers, organisms such as yeast, Group B streptococci, coliforms, *Staphylococcus aureus*, and various anaerobes may be present. Although so close to this pool of microbes, the uterus is generally absent of bacteria, which attests to the efficiency of the cervix as a barrier. The proximity of the vagina to the anus, given the structure of the female genital site, ensures that many females will at some time have their vaginal microbial flora containing some fecal organism whether in large or small quantitation.

Given these aforementioned descriptions of normal flora, it is not surprising to see why infection is so common. We live in **symbiosis** with our usual microbial flora, but given the opportunity, many of them can create harm in the right environment. The likelihood for these bacteria to infect is then a function of the individual traits of a given bacterium and the likelihood that it will be present at the time that an opportunity arises. Given the presence of such microbes, it is also not difficult to see that transmission from person to person will occur frequently during routine contacts; an alteration of behaviour that increases contact or increases the presence of bacteria on less typical sites (e.g., poor hygiene) will potentially enhance communicability, while strict attention to cleanliness (e.g., handwashing) will likely be associated with lesser sharing of bacteria from normal flora.

Do alterations in the quantity or make-up of the normal microbial flora lead to disease states? The answer is a resounding YES! For example, antibiotic use, which may suppress some normally-present bacteria, could lead to an inbalance whereby antibiotic resistance microbes flourish. Yeast infections are a common example of the latter as in thrush (oral candidiasis) or yeast vaginitis. Another form of vaginal disease, termed bacterial vaginosis, may result from an overgrowth of anaerobes relative to the predominant lactobacilli. This latter change is associated with a shift in vaginal acidity (usually ~pH 3-4) which may be a marker for the disease. Marked suppression of large bowel microbes may lead to proliferation of *Clostridium difficile* which in large numbers may produce sufficient quantities of toxin to result in diarrhea ("antibiotic associated colitis"). During some virus infections of the respiratory tract, the environment of the nose becomes conducive to the overgrowth of *Streptococcus pneumoniae* and *Haemophilius influenzae* which are more virulent than other mouth bacteria. If there are underlying medical conditions which impede the motility of the gastrointestinal tract, large numbers of bacteria may be present in the small bowel which could lead to malabsorption.

Overall, the presence of usual microbial flora is both a necessity and a hazard. Infection can arise from either these endogenous microbes or from microbes which are acquired from some external focus.

Protecting Itself

Does the body live in a microbial world or do microbes live in a human world? Either way, it is obvious that we must have numerous ways in which we can cope with and survive from the potential of microbes. Indeed, the body is complete with many protective features (Table 1).

Foremost among these protective mechanisms is the basic anatomy of the body with its usual structural barriers (i.e., skin and mucous membrane). Skin has numerous layers which must breached. The areas which harbour large quantities of normal microbial flora (i.e., nose, throat, gastrointestinal tract, and vagina), all have a similarly layered anatomic barrier called the **mucous membrane**. Burns present a major interruption of the skin which makes infection more probable. Invasive medical and dental procedures and the presence of transcutaneous devices (e.g., venous access lines) are other common examples of how these anatomic barriers are interrupted. The central nervous system is quite uncommonly infected, and this is not surprising given that there are several barriers that microbes must overcome in order to gain entry.

The body has its own cleansing methods which continue uninterrupted in a healthy state twenty-four hours a day. The gastrointestinal tract is normally motile with waves of ring-like contractions which move towards the terminal end (peristalsis). These motions serve to propel food and bacteria onwards. The mouth and gastrointestinal tract produce secretions (e.g., saliva, mucous) which act in part to lavage the sites. Tears which are produced continually from lacrimal glands serve to wash the eye's surface. The respiratory tract is for the most part lined with cells that have cilia. Cilia extend into the lumina of the respiratory tract and exist as very tiny hair-like projections which beat in a whip-like fashion towards the mouth and, in doing so, clear bacteria which are accidentally aspirated from saliva. Urine from the bladder serves in part to flush the urethra. Interruptions of these cleansing mechanisms are each associated with greater susceptibility to infection at the respective site.

The body's inherent reflexes have a role in protection. There is a natural reflex to gag or swallow when the back of the throat is contacted. Without this reflex, food and saliva might be inadvertently aspirated and thereby increase the opportunity for pneumonia. Coughing and sneezing also participate in clearing the airways; suppression of cough by the use of antitussive medications may at times worsen a lower respiratory tract infection. The automaticity of the bladder ensures routine expulsion of urine which, if present in a stagnant bladder, can accommodate infection. The normal tone of the anal sphincter ensures prevention of untimely soilage of the perineal area.

Table 1. Defence mechanisms of the body.

A. Body's response to stress
    a)   fever
    b)   emesis
    c)   diarrhea
    d)   bladder contraction

B. Normal reflexes
    a)   gag reflex of mouth
    b)   coughing
    c)   sneezing
    d)   bladder automaticity
    e)   continence of the anal sphincter

C. Normal anatomic barriers
    a)   skin
    b)   mucous membranes
    c)   conjunctivae of eyes
    d)   ear drum

D. Normal cleansing mechanisms and body secretions
    a)   tears and salivary glands
    b)   intestinal secretory enzymes (e.g., digestive enzymes)
    c)   intestinal bile
    d)   cilia of the respiratory tract cells
    e)   peristalsis in the gastrointestinal tract
    f)   stomach acidity
    g)   vaginal acidity

E. Usual microbial flora of the body

F. Genetic variation of the body and its influence on responses to infection and on the structure of receptors for microbial attachment

G. Immunity
    a)   antibody
        -   systemic
        -   mucosal
    b)   cell-mediated responses
    c)   cells that engulf microbes
    d)   inflammation and mediators of inflammation

H. Human knowledge and human capability

Normal chemical extremes or enzyme production can affect microbes. As previously detailed, both stomach and vaginal acidities are protective. Apart from providing a cleansing effect, tears and saliva have digestive enzymes (e.g., lysozyme) which can break down the cell wall of Gram positive bacteria especially. In the upper small bowel, the bile duct injects bile which has been produced by the liver and which is stored by the gallbladder. Bile is quite active as an antimicrobial agent against many bacteria. Pancreatic juices which are also entering the small bowel lumen may have an effect on the surface structures and cell wall of microbes.

The body's mechanical response to the stress of infection, although more a consequence of disease, may have an indirect protective role. For example, both diarrhea and vomiting expulse noxious bacteria and their products. Infection of the bladder will often cause cramping and increased frequency of contraction. In many ways, fever may have a beneficial effect on infection.

The initiation of infection often requires a direct and active linkage between the microbe and sites of uptake or infection as we have previously discussed. The human side of this initiation is called the **receptor** which will extend from cells as either a protein, a complex sugar molecule, or a combination of these and other structures. Receptors for different microbes may be quite variable in their makeup. This receptor however may have a variable structure, and variability which is dependent on the genetic makeup of an individual can lead to differences in the affinity of the germ to the human cell. Therefore, inherent genetic variability among humans may make them more or less susceptible to infection.

The **immune system** is a complex collection of protective mechanisms which must have evolved to directly search and destroy intruders (i.e., microbes). This system has an innate ability to protect the body without ever having previously seen the germ. In addition, the immune system can evolve to create new defence tactics when it has had some exposure to the microbe. We will discuss these functions shortly.

The aforementioned defence mechanisms are invaluable, and they provide a balance that is sufficient for the majority of human-microbial interactions. Nevertheless, the next level of protection is scientific innovation which provides antibiotics and vaccines for us. That is, the human mind, through its ability to understand and problem solve, provides in contemporary times an important defence. It may be that microbes have been on earth longer than humans and that they have enormous potential for change and to adapt. Our ability to strategize provides a counter-balance. The complex human central nervous system is an underestimated defence mechanism. On one hand, we might assume that advanced science will be the major component of human knowledge which contributes to prevention. To the contrary, it is very simple concepts such as handwashing or hygienic food preparation that have the most to contribute. The latter are no less a function, however, of human capability.

An Immunology Primer

Immunology is the study of the body's defences as they are developed to recognize existing and new structures (the "immune system"). As we have detailed previously, the body has a number of defence mechanisms which are consistent and not induced. **Immunity**, however, is developmental and dynamic. As the fetus develops and the body grows, they are in need of recognizing and differentiating self and non-self. Self-antigens (an antigen can be thought of as the simplest of structural forms that may be recognized by the immune response) cannot be attacked. Otherwise, survival would be a problem at the earliest stages. Non-self antigens, however, are considerably variable, and because they are foreign and generally different from structures of the body, they are perceived by the body as something that should be responded to. This response, however, complicated or simple as it may be, in large part is a reflection of the "immune response" (Figure 2). There are three components of immune responses that are generally recognized. The first of these is the antibody response (scientifically termed the '**humoral immune response**') which consists of proteins produced in response to stimuli by specific types of cells. The second of these is immunity that is conferred by a number of (immune) cells directly. The latter do not produce antibody but are capable of providing a direct form of resistance to infection by actively playing a part in the recognition of and in the fight against infection. Lastly, in addition to antibody and infection-directed cells, there are products of cells that are affected by infection, cells which are at the site of infection, and other naturally existing factors which are able to modulate the overall response to infection.

   Antibody-producing cells (**lymphocytes**: a form of white blood cell) are present throughout most parts of the body but are especially concentrated in areas which are highly exposed to germs and infection. Therefore, there are many antibody-producing cells which exist along mucous membranes (e.g., gut, nose, mouth) where germs normally reside and where many infections are initiated. Antibody-producing cells are common in blood. Lymph nodes are essentially concentrations of immune cells which include numerous antibody-producing cells; the size of lymph nodes may increase with response to a local infection as cells replicate in response or as they may have immune cells from other sites that migrate to this centre. The system of antibody-producing cells is considerably complex since it needs to be able to respond to a large number of infections

Figure 2. 'Arms' of the human immune response.

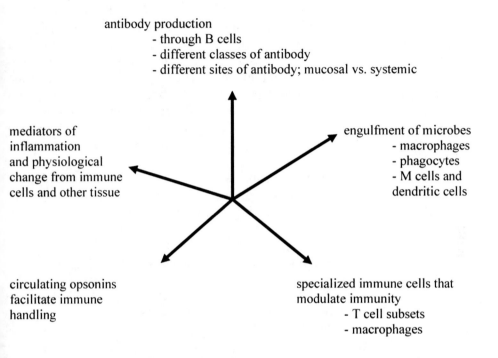

antibody production
- through B cells
- different classes of antibody
- different sites of antibody; mucosal vs. systemic

mediators of
inflammation
and physiological
change from immune
cells and other tissue

engulfment of microbes
- macrophages
- phagocytes
- M cells and
dendritic cells

circulating opsonins
facilitate immune
handling

specialized immune cells that
modulate immunity
- T cell subsets
- macrophages

and foreign materials. Antibody-producing cells are migratory and may home in to the areas of infection. These cells will replicate in order to provide a sufficient supply of needed antibody.

Antibodies are complex proteins that have the ability to recognize and attack the foreign structures (Figure 3). For example, antibodies may specifically recognize the attachment filaments of bacteria or the coat structure of a virus. Antibodies are developed in response to a complex event whereby the foreign structure is recognized by a specialized cell, which then presents the structure in such a way to turn on the antibody-producing cell. Antibody recognition of a particular structure is very specific. When the antibody binds to the structures so recognized, the resulting complex may inactivate the germ or at least hinder its function. In addition, the complex of antibody and structure (also termed **antigen**) may be able to initiate a number a secondary events which further inactivates the germ or perhaps recruit more forms of the immune response. Antibodies (also termed **immunoglobulins**) take the form of slightly different structures (Table 2). Immunoglobulin M is a complex antibody which is the first to develop in response to a new infection antigen. Immunoglobulin G follows the latter response and remains in the body for longer term protection. Immunoglobulin A is most important in immune responses at mucosal surfaces. It is recognized that there are literally grams of antibody being produced by the body's immune cells daily. Much of the antibody remains circulating in a person's blood, but antibody (especially immunoglobulin A) can be actively excreted into the mucosal sites. It is believed that antibody-producing cells in one part of the body are capable of migrating to other areas of the body given an appropriate stimulus (e.g., infection). After antibodies are produced, they may continue to be produced at low levels thereafter. This lingering antibody may serve to provide full or partial protection against the germ for a short period of time or even indefinitely.

Infection-fighting immune cells which do not produce antibody are several. There are non-specifically targeted cells called **polymorphonuclear cells** (or **phagocytes**; another form of white blood cell) which ingest foreign

Figure 3. Schematic diagram of an antibody (immunoglobulin) molecule.

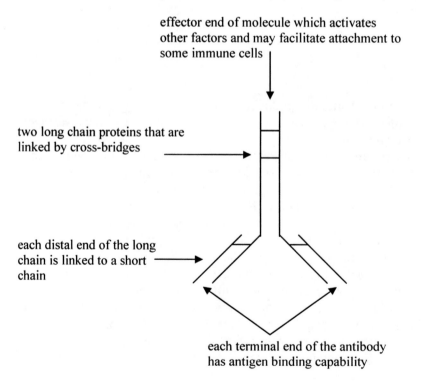

effector end of molecule which activates other factors and may facilitate attachment to some immune cells

two long chain proteins that are linked by cross-bridges

each distal end of the long chain is linked to a short chain

each terminal end of the antibody has antigen binding capability

Table 2. Types of human antibody.

Immunoglobulin G (IgG)
- single molecular form (as in Figure 3)
- different types of IgG occur – IgG1, IgG2, IgG3, IgG4
- most plentiful antibody in circulating blood (over one gram for every 100 ml. of blood; ~80% of total serum antibody)
- over 30 gm./d. synthesized by body
- activates microbial killing activity
- binds to phagocytic cells and increases their activity
- crosses the placenta from mother to fetus
- basis for most protective antibody in the body
- has a long secondary response after initial infection

Immunoglobulin M (IgM)
- composed of 5 single antibody molecules that are linked together
- occurs as an initial response to infection but wanes thereafter
- may reoccur after repeated exposure to the same pathogen but not to the same extent as IgG
- can activate some microbial killing activities
- can be a marker for recent active infection

Immunoglobulin A (IgA)
- exists as either single or double molecular forms
- two types exist: IgA1, IgA2
- can activate some microbial lytic activity
- important for protection at mucosal sites but also circulates in the body

Immunoglobulin E (IgE)
- binds to cells that mediate allergic responses
- has other roles in allergic responses
- can be a marker for allergy to certain substances

Immunoglobulin D (IgD)
- single molecular form
- mainly immune cell-associated
- functions not apparently as diverse as other antibodies

particles and attempt to digest them after engulfing the foreign particles and having taken them internally to meet the cell's degradative enzymes. This form of response can take place throughout the body. Phagocytes will be recruited to a site of infection and a collection of them gives rise to "**pus**". Variations of these cells, called **eosinophils**, may especially be involved in immune responses to parasites; eosinophils release chemicals which lead to an allergic response. There are other germ-engulfing cells throughout the body. The direction of these latter cells to the site of infection may involve stimulation from other immune cells (non-antibody producing lymphocytes). The presence of the foreign antigen will stimulate the latter cells which in turn will signal chemicals that draw germ-engulfing cells to the site of need. Some of these non-antibody producing cells may also be capable of destroying the body's own cells which may have been infected. For example, a virus has invaded a body cell and will replicate within. As the immune cells may not be able to enter the body cell to directly attack the virus, the immune cell will destroy the entire cell itself thereby attacking the virus and all! When groups of antibody non-producing cells work together to achieve the common goal of recognizing and destroying infection, we term this phenomenon "**cell-mediated immunity**". The Mantoux test, which is a skin test for tuberculosis and which is manifest as an area of skin redness and elevation when positive, is but a measure of cell-mediated immunity to a purified protein derivative of the tuberculosis germ (*Mycobacterium tuberculosis*).

When cells and tissues of the body are infected, many of them are capable of releasing or stimulating the production of chemicals or signal products (**cytokines**) which further the response to infection. These agents can increase inflammation, call for help to immune cells which are residing elsewhere, or directly interact with the infecting germs. When immune cells are called to the site of infection, they too may release signal molecules to further call other immune cells. They too may also release products which affect the local milieu (e.g., increasing blood circulation to the area; e.g., increasing inflammation). There may also be naturally circulating factors (e.g., opsonins, complement) which are antibacterial; they may act in consort with antibody to inactivate the invading pathogen.

It is evident that the body has many potential responses to infection. Not all infections, however, stimulate the same type or sequence of responses. Most typical bacterial causes of infection lead to a migration of phagocytes to the area of infection as an initial response. This response will be followed by antibody-producing cells. Viruses, although potentially leading to a recruitment of the same to a lesser degree, will especially invite the cell-mediated immune system. There are many exceptions, and in the end, the body elaborates a response depending on the type of pathogen, the site of infection, and its previous experience if any with the same infection.

As we understand the many different aspects of the immune system, we will by default understand how defects or absences of any of these may lead to the **"immunodeficiency"** state. When cancer patients are given chemotherapy to destroy a malignancy, these same pharmaceutical agents may inadvertently destroy some of the helpful immune cells, thereby reducing the host defences. When a child is born with a defect in phagocytic cell function, the child thereafter will be susceptible to infections which are best prevented or stopped by these cells. Defects in the immune system may include one or many of these protective mechanisms. The immune system and non-immune host defences collectively serve as the balance in nature to the many opportunities that germs have to infect.

Food For Thought

1. For a microbe that must enter the large bowel (that is, the terminal portion of the alimentary canal) to attach and then cause an infection (e.g., diarrhea), consider the needs and obstacles for this process to occur.
2. How does the normal human microbial flora provide benefit to the host?
3. Apart from viruses, what types of microbes are able to enter cells rather than simply cause an infection outside of cells?
4. How might the protective immune system response to toxin-producing microbes differ from the protective immune response to microbes that are invasive?

Supplemental Reading

Abbas AK, Lichtman AH. *Basic Immunology*. 3rd Edition. Philadelphia, PA:Saunders Elsevier, 2011.
- concise but advanced text

Delves PJ, Martin SJ, Burton DR, Roitt IM. *Roitt's Essential Immunology*. Oxford, UK:Blackwell Publishing Ltd., 2006.
- presenting essentials in a colourful manner

Larsen B. Vaginal flora in health and disease. *Clinical Obstetrics and Gynecology* Vol. 36:pages 107-121 (1993).
- a review paper from a medical journal which exemplifies the role of usual human microbial flora in health and disease. The relevance of this paper is unchanged for today.

Lee YK, Salminen S. *Handbook of Probiotics and Prebiotics*. 2nd Edition. New York, NY:Wiley, 2009.

- an interesting concept of restoring or modifying normal human flora in order to maintain or restore health

Levinson S. *Review of Medical Microbiology and Immunology.* 11th Edition. New York, NY:McGraw-Hill, 2010.
- concise and to the point

"Where the telescope ends, the microscope begins.
Which of the two has the grander view?"
                    Victor Hugo
                    Les Misérables, 1862

IV. Diagnosis Facilitates Prevention

The control and prevention of infection are dependent on the knowledge of what we are dealing with and what we should anticipate. It is only natural therefore that the laboratory must play an integral role in these endeavours. Clinical diagnoses which are dependent on a patient's history and physical findings will often provide the best guess for an illness, although some infections will be accompanied by classic symptoms and signs. Nevertheless, the definitive understanding of infection often requires an appreciation of the clinical illness along with more definitive laboratory support. A laboratory's capabilities are many, and the diagnostic request must follow a logical sequence of what is most likely.

If a laboratory is to impact on infection control, its tools must be accurate and then be provided on a timely basis. The diagnostic test will most often confirm clinical suspicions and less commonly give clues to less likely causes. The course of some infections may be altered by antibiotics or vaccines such that further spread may be prevented. In addition to defining an active infection, the laboratory test may be needed to screen a patient population which carries the germ asymptomatically or while latently infected. Some diagnostic tools (e.g., antibody determination) may determine whether a patient's body has previously acquired knowledge of immunity. The latter may be critical to the health care worker as well. Diagnostic procedures may find the unexpected. Insights may be gathered when novel infectious agents are discovered.

Non-Specific Diagnostics

Laboratory techniques which may assist in the diagnosis of infection are many. In addition to microbe-specific methods, there are a number of relatively non-specific indicators which may be used in various circumstances. These diagnostic tests, when evaluated in combination with clinical features of the illness, may be sufficient to provide a conclusive diagnosis. Microbe-specific assays may or may not be used as an adjunct. Table 1 illustrates some of these non-specific diagnostics and some of the circumstances in which they are of some value. In general, these assessments determine variations that have been associated with a particular illness and which are outside of normal physiological range. The indicator may be highly suggestive that a particular illness exists (e.g., marked increase in blood lymphocyte number during active whooping cough), or a particular organ is affected (e.g., liver enzyme increase in blood signifying hepatitis of some sort). The number of non-specific tests which maybe used to investigate a given illness may be few or many. As well, it may be that only a specific diagnostic test will be required.

Table 1. Examples of applications for non-specific diagnostics.

index being measured	implication
increased white blood cell count	inflammatory process
increased white blood cell count in which 'neutrophil' subcount is increased	presumptively a bacterial infection
increased erythrocyte sedimentation rate (ESR)	inflammatory process
increased white blood cell count in which 'eosinophil' subcount is markedly increased	possibly systemic parasite infection (or allergic reaction)
markedly suppressed white blood cell count in a newborn	possibly systemic bacterial infection
increased C reactive protein	inflammatory process
increased circulating liver enzyme profile indicative of liver cell damage (e.g., ALT or AST)	hepatitis
increased white blood cells in the urine	possible urinary tract infection
specific electrocardiogram changes	myocarditis (heart inflammation)
specific abnormalities in x-ray exams or similar tests	may be suggestive of infection (e.g., chest X-ray signs of pneumonia)

Microbe-Specific Measures

As the microbial world is complex, so too is the science which has led to the discovery and diagnosis of the many infectious diseases for which we are at risk. There are a variety of laboratory tools which exist, and the use of any particular form of testing procedure will very much depend on the specific organism being considered, the infection status, or the sign of infection being observed. Given the great complexity of germ and host response, there is no single test by which all infections can be determined. The specific methods for any given infection therefore need to be learned or assessed at the appropriate time.

We must be reminded that diagnostic tests are only one part of the process. The physician or health care worker must appreciate fully a patient's history and complaints. In many circumstances, an examination of the patient is equally relevant. Given the latter, the caregiver must come to a best guess among very equally or lesser possibilities; the laboratory test then acts to provide more accuracy when required in addition to the aforementioned non-specific diagnostics.

Microbe-specific measures will basically consist of direct detection of the germ at the site of the specific infection by the finding of the germ itself, a special component of the germ, or by a measurable specific effect of the micro-organism. Alternatively, infection may be determined by the demonstration of an immune response to the microbe (i.e., an infection will have given rise to immunity and therefore a measure of immunity implies infection). For a given infection, a single diagnostic test may suffice; in other circumstances, combinations of diagnostic tests may be required. The following methods of microbe-specific tests are used more or less:

microscopy and **staining** - from a tissue or fluid sample
culture - growth of the microbe by artificial means in the laboratory
serology- showing an immune response
antigen detection - only parts of the microbe ("antigens") are detected
bioactivity - a biological effect of the microbe is present in a tissue or fluid as demonstrated in the laboratory
genetic detection - microbial DNA or RNA is detected in the clinical specimen

Microscopy and Staining

Although many infections may be defined by the demonstration of microbial growth in the clinical specimen, these culture techniques are occasionally hampered by a time delay to positivity. This time delay is measured in days to weeks depending on the specific etiological agent. The clinical diagnosis may occasionally be accurate at the time a patient is seen, but there are many circumstances where a more timely laboratory-assisted diagnosis is more desirable. Given the potential delay for culture methods, the finding of the organism at the site of infection by a microscopic method has the potential to facilitate rapid diagnosis. In some circumstances, the microbe cannot be cultivated on a practical basis, and therefore, a direct microscopic method may be the only useful approach (Table 2).

Staining techniques are many, and they will vary depending on the size and nature of the microbe. A stain is essentially a tool to highlight the microbe while differentiating it from the background of human tissue (i.e., the clinical sample). The stain may also be capable of illustrating the differences among various microbes. There are many different types of staining techniques, and they may be used for different forms of microscopy.

The most common form of microscopy is **light microscopy**, with which

Table 2. Examples of non-cultivable microbes or microbes that are not usually cultured.

microbe	disease	preferred diagnostic method
Treponema pallidum	syphilis	serodiagnosis or microscopy
rickettsiae	several variable illnesses	not routinely cultivated; serodiagnosis or genetic detection
borreliae	Lyme disease, relapsing fever	not routinely cultivated; serodiagnosis or genetic detection
Tropheryma whippelii	Whipple's disease	genetic detection
enteric parasites	several variable illnesses	microscopy of stool or genetic detection
Plasmodium species	malaria	microscopy of blood
hepatitis C/hepatitis B	hepatitis	serodiagnosis or antigen detection or genetic detection
arboviruses	several variable illnesses	not routinely cultured; serodiagnosis or genetic detection

most individuals are familiar as the standard form of microscopic examination (Figures 1 and 2). Most bacteria, fungi, and parasites can be seen with this tool, but viruses are not. Therefore, standard microscopy will usually be unable to determine the presence of a virus in a respiratory tract sampling from a patient with a cold. Two more-widely used examples for standard light microscopy and staining are the **Gram stain** and the **Ziehl-Neelsen** stain. The Gram stain is especially used for demonstrating bacteria and common yeast. The Gram stain can determine differences based on characteristics such as color, shape, and distribution. "**Gram positive**" bacteria will appear purple under the microscope while "**Gram negative**" bacteria will appear pink or red. Shape may vary from circular (**coccus**; plural - cocci) to rod-shaped (**bacillus**; plural - bacilli) to curved. Different bacterial groups will be typically of one Gram stain color and shape (see Figures 12 a and b of Chapter II). On a strict laboratory basis, the Gram stain will be useful to the laboratory worker who will use this technique (completed in approximately 5-10 minutes) to differentiate among bacteria that have grown on artificial media. Of further value, the Gram stain may be used to rapidly identify the presence of an unlikely category of bacteria which are actively causing infection (Table 3). For example, a swab may be obtained from a post-surgical wound of a female who has undergone elective Caesarian section for the birth of her child. The finding of Gram positive cocci in clusters from a

Figure 1. Photograph of the light microscope.

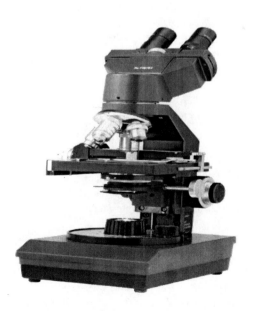

Figure 2. Line drawing of the light microscope function.

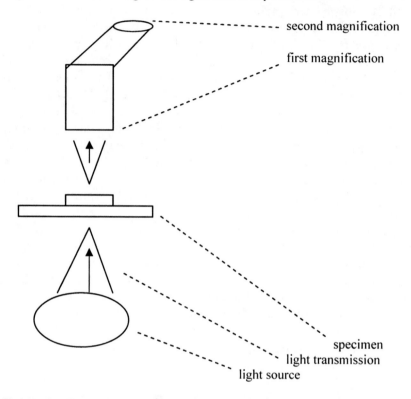

Table 3. Examples of Gram stain patterns in clinical specimens and their implications for clinical practice.

specimen	Gram stain appearance	implication
urethral swab from male	Gram negative diplococci and white blood cells	*Neisseria gonorrhoeae* as a cause of a sexually transmitted disease
cerebrospinal fluid	Gram negative diplococci Gram negative coccobacilli Gram positive diplococci	*Neisseria meningitidis* *Haemophilus influenzae* *Streptococcus pneumoniae*
tissue from gangrene	Gram positive bacilli	*Clostridium* species
tissue from necrotizing fasciitis	Gram positive cocci in chains	*Streptococcus pyogenes*

Gram stain of a swab which is subsequently smeared on a microscope slide will indicate with reasonable probability that the causative agent is *Staphylococcus aureus*. Apart from actively knowing of the bacterial cause, this best guess will influence decision-making regarding the antibiotic which should be used given that the different antibiotics will be used preferentially for different microbes. The Gram stain will have provided this information within minutes, whereas the culture identification of the bacterium will require a minimum of another day at best. The Ziehl-Neelsen stain (also known as the **"acid fast stain"**) is particularly employed to find bacteria which are the cause of tuberculosis (mycobacteria, particularly *Mycobacterium tuberculosis*). A 'silver stain' is used to specifically highlight *Pneumocystis jirovecii* in respiratory specimens (a cause of unusual pneumonia in immune compromised patients).

Another form of microscopy that may be used in special circumstances is **fluorescence microscopy**. Here, the microbes in the clinical sample are tagged with a specific antibody that is purposely joined to a substance which is fluorescent under ultraviolet light. The antibody has been purposely designed to be specific to the germ of interest. The fluorescence microscope, in contrast to the light microscope, is able to allow ultraviolet light exposure of the microscope slide, as well as the visualization of the purposely-labelled fluorescent germ. The structure of the microscope is similar to the light microscope except that the specimen is exposed to fluorescent light which is then seen through a series of special filters. This technique might be used to illustrate individual organisms or perhaps large clusters of microbes within human cells (e.g., for viruses). Fluorescence microscopy will especially be used when light microscopy and usual stains are not sufficiently helpful. Indeed, some bacteria will not stain at all with the more routine Gram stain technique. Table 4 gives examples where fluorescent microscopy may be used.

The electron microscope is a bulky instrument, uncommonly used, and for the purposes of infection, used essentially only to detect viruses in special circumstances. It will magnify much more than other forms of microscopy.

Microbial Culture

Although the identification of a microbe by the staining of a clinical sample may give valuable clinical confirmation, it may not be sufficiently complete. One may actually multiply the microbe in the laboratory directly; this is referred to as **'culture'**. With this process, the microbe can be exactly identified, and it may be multiplied to the basic minimum that will be needed for assessing antimicrobial susceptibility. If culture is to be attempted, the clinical specimen or swab must be transported to the laboratory appropriately. It must not have been exposed to

Table 4. Examples for the use of fluorescence microscopy in medical microbiology.

1. Detection of antibodies for serodiagnostic purposes.

2. Detection of *Treponema pallidum* (cause of syphilis) directly in clinical swab smears from genital ulcers.

3. Confirmation of particular bacteria or viruses that are cultured in the laboratory.

4. Direct detection of virus-infected cells (e.g., herpes simplex lesions; e.g., virus respiratory infections).

5. Direct detection of *Bordetella pertussis* or *Legionella* species in respiratory secretions.

extremes of the environment (e.g., drying or excess temperature). Transport containers with balanced salt solutions and stabilizers may provide protection for specimen transfer. Transport containers and solutions will vary depending on the nature of the infecting agent. Table 5 details some specific transport needs.

Once received in the laboratory, growth will be attempted on solid or liquid media depending on the specimen and the microbe to be grown. The specific samples to be obtained and assessed are dependent on the sites of infection (Table 6). Whereas some infections may involve a single site sampling (e.g., throat swab for a sore throat), others may mandate several samplings which can include an assessment for different types of microbes. The various subgroups of microbes may be cultured by different techniques. Bacteria are commonly cultured in 24-48 hours on solid and liquid culture media. The solid media allow for growth of '**bacterial colonies**'; the liquid or 'broth' media allow for enrichment of few to many organisms. Some bacteria may require extended periods of growth, up to weeks and possibly months (e.g., causes of tuberculosis require several weeks). Fungi will take many days to weeks; yeast forms often require only a few days. Viruses require many days to weeks with few exceptions but are more temperamental due to the need to grow them in mammalian cells. It is generally difficult to grow parasites, and thus microscopic methods are usually used for parasite examination.

As we will understand, the microbial world is complex; this diversity has led to varying requirements for microbial culture. For bacteria alone, knowledge in regards to culture methods is considerable. Unfortunately, these issues place demands on the health care worker, especially physicians, to be fully cognizant of the particular needs for each infectious agent and/or site of infection.

Table 5. Transport requirements for specific microbes.

Routine bacteria	- balanced salt solutions with or without gel; anaerobic bacteria may require special transport
Viruses	- balanced salt solution with a protein buffer and with antibacterial antibiotics
Chlamydia species	- as above but a different mixture of antibiotics; culture has largely been replaced by non-culture methods
Bordetella pertussis	- charcoal-based media; requirements for specimens that are to be used for molecular diagnostics may be different
Neisseria gonorrhoeae	- charcoal-based swabs yield higher culture yields

Table 6. Examples of common infections and samples which may be acquired for diagnostic purposes.

Infections	Specimens
Urinary tract infections	urine sent for bacterial culture; quantitative counts of bacteria are required in addition to defining presence of pathogens
Gastroenteritis	freshly voided stool specimen submitted
Meningitis	cerebrospinal fluid submitted
Pneumonia	coughed sputum submitted
Blood-borne bacterial infections	blood submitted in blood culture bottles
Sore throat, wound infections, conjunctivitis	swabs from sites are submitted in transport media
Virus infections	specimens from direct sites of infection
Intestinal parasites	stool sent in a specific formalin fixative or equivalent

Serology

Serology (**serodiagnosis**) generally refers to the technology which allows the laboratory to determine whether a humoral immune (**antibody**) response has occurred as result of infection as we have previously detailed (see Chapter III). The body's immune system recognizes a foreign substance and then directs an antibody response. The finding of an immune response then implies that the body has been infected. Also as previously stated, different types of antibodies may be produced. IgM antibody generally results as a consequence of new infections, and IgG antibody follows. Measurement of antibody during early infection may be compared to a measurement from late in infection; an increment of certain proportions between the two measures may be indicative of a recent infection having occurred. We refer to these changes as '**seroconversion**'.

The finding of IgM which is directed to a microbe is often an indication of recent infection. Usually the latter antibodies wane over several weeks to months. IgG antibody tends to persist, however, for many months to many years depending on the intensity of the response to the infection. Therefore, if one were only able to detect IgG antibodies to a microbe, their presence might simply reflect past exposure and not necessarily acute infection. Some microbes may cause recurrent infection, and it may be valuable to detect a relative increase in IgG over several days to weeks. The latter approach may often only serve of retrospective value. For infections where a medical intervention may be of value (e.g., antibiotic treatment), a more rapid form of diagnosis may be desirable if available. In certain circumstances where culture of the microbe is delayed or impossible, timely serodiagnosis may still prove of value.

There are many different ways by which serological tests can be performed, and these often prove confusing to the novice. Table 7 and associated Figures 3-7 exemplify this diversity. Again one must keep in mind that all are essentially assessments of antibody response, regardless of the variation and technical method (i.e., one has the antigen already prepared in the laboratory, and one determines whether there is an antibody response to it).

Due to the technical methods which are employed for antibody detection, problems occasionally arise with the indirect methods whereby the assessment may be non-specific or in error. Immunoblotting is quite specific, and therefore the results are somewhat more definitive. Given these difficulties, it may be that the more indirect test will be used to screen for infection, especially since these are more easily performed. Immunoblotting, which is more tedious and more difficult to perform on many samples simultaneously, is occasionally used as a more definitive and confirmatory test. As an example, antibodies to HIV (Human Immunodeficiency Virus) as a marker for infection will often be determined by an enzyme immunoassay which is a reasonably sensitive test. Since the possibility of being wrong, especially falsely positive, has tremendous medical and psychosocial implications, a confirmatory immunoblotting test (also known as the 'Western Blot '), which is specific, will also be performed.

Table 7. Methods for the detection of antibody.

Agglutination - serum (a component of blood which contains antibody in part) is mixed with antigen. Antigen -antibody interactions are determined visually by the unaided eye (Figure 3).

Immunofluorescence Assay - serum is mixed with antigen. The antigen-antibody complex is visualized with the aid of another antibody which binds to the microbe-specific human antibody and which is tagged or labelled with a fluorescent marker (Figure 4).

Complement Fixation Test - serum antibody-antigen reaction is determined by the activation of another serum protein called complement which binds to the antigen antibody complex (Figure 5).

Enzyme Immunoassay - also termed ELISA, EIA, or enzyme-linked immunosorbent assay. The antigen-antibody interaction is indirectly detected by another antibody which is labelled with an enzyme that converts a colourless to a coloured compound (Figure 6).

Immunoblotting - a more direct method in which antibody reactivity to specific antigens can be determined in contrast to the indirect detection methods above. The antigen needs to be highly purified and resolved for this method (Figure 7).

Figure 3. Agglutination reaction applied to serological diagnosis.

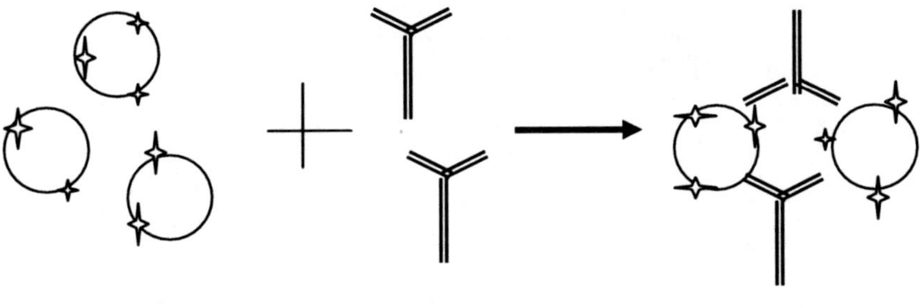

| antigen-coated carrier particles | antibody present in serum sample | agglutination of antigen and antibody |

82

Figure 4. Immunofluorescence assay for the detection of antibody.

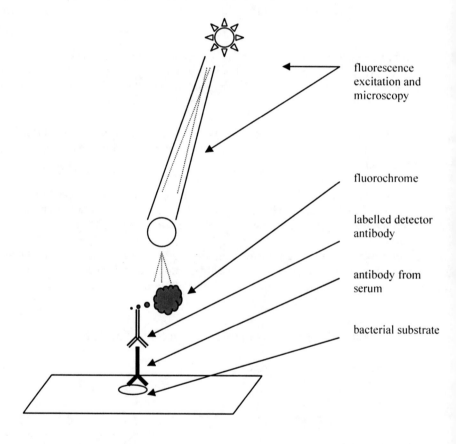

fluorescence
excitation and
microscopy

fluorochrome

labelled detector
antibody

antibody from
serum

bacterial substrate

Figure 5. The complement fixation test and its use for detecting the presence of antigen-specific antibody.

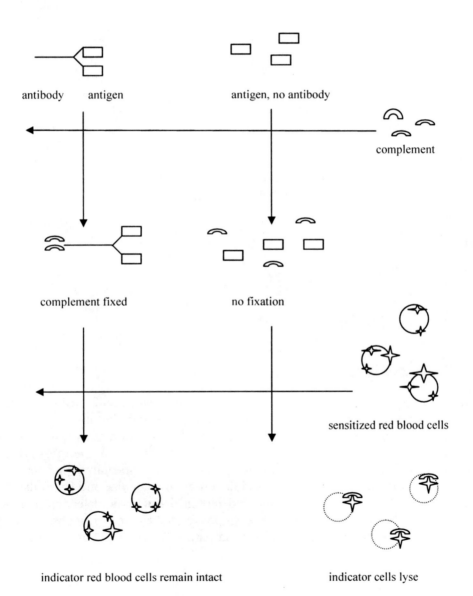

antibody   antigen

antigen, no antibody

complement

complement fixed

no fixation

sensitized red blood cells

indicator red blood cells remain intact

indicator cells lyse

Figure 6. Enzyme-linked immunosorbent assay for the detection of antibodies.

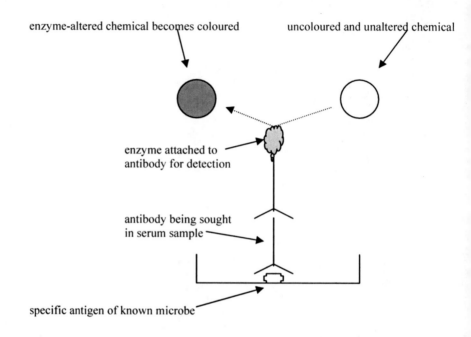

<u>Antigen Detection</u>

If one has the ability to either grow, or otherwise isolate wholly or in part some of the components of the microbe in question, one may be able to use these substances (**antigens**) to immunize animals. That is, the antigen given to the animal as an immunization may allow the development of microbe-directed antibodies. Once these antibodies are produced experimentally, they may be harvested from the animal's blood and then used to recognize antigen in the test. Therefore, whereas serology uses a predetermined antigen to detect an antibody response, antigen detection uses a known pre-formed antibody response to detect the presence of the microbe, wholly or in part. In principle, therefore, serology and antigen detection are converse.

Figure 7. An example of an immunoblot for confirmatory serodiagnostic testing. The test antigen of the microbe is broken down and components of it are separated onto a solid support by chemical and electrical means. Antibody source (serum) and detector antibody are incubated with this resolved antigen, and the presence of antibody is identified by discrete linear colour changes. Thus, multiple positive bands of reaction are indicative of multiple antibodies present which are directed to different components of the microbe. The strength of the apparent linear antibody response depends on the amount of antibody available.

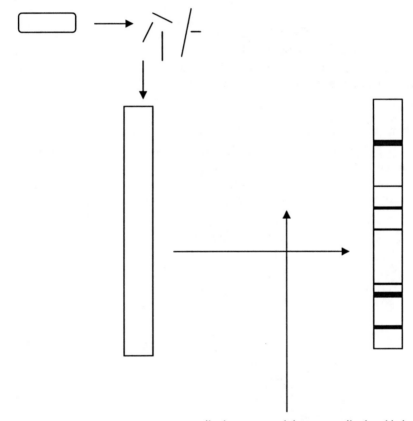

serum antibody source and detector antibody added

Antigen detection can be applied directly to a clinical specimen, and it has the potential to yield a quicker result, in part due to the lack of dependency on a serological response which may require many days from the onset of infection. This technique is currently useful for a limited number of infections and for a limited number of body sites and samples.

The technical jargon of antigen detection techniques is somewhat similar to serodiagnosis and includes: agglutination, immunofluorescence, enzyme immunoassay, and radioimmunoassay (Figure 8).

Bioactivity

Rather than directly detecting antigen or determining the occurrence of an immune response, it may be possible to demonstrate that a microbe is present in a given body site by the finding of a biological response or activity that may be directly attributable to a microbial component.

Figure 8. Example of the configuration for a radioimmunoassay for antigen detection. Essentially, the reaction is similar to an enzyme immunoassay, but the detector antibody is labelled with a radioactive chemical. The antigen is first captured with an antibody. The amount of antigen is thus proportionate to the amount of radioactive material that remains and is measured.

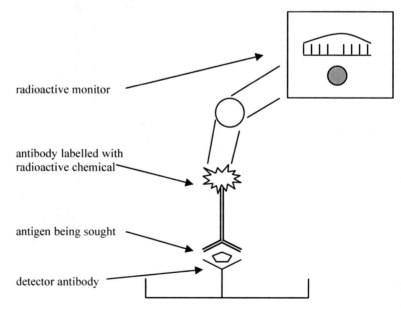

radioactive monitor

antibody labelled with radioactive chemical

antigen being sought

detector antibody

There are several examples of how this may be applied, but the following two examples serve well. *Clostridium botulinum* causes botulism via toxin production. The infection is suspected by the finding of bacterial toxin in food or in the victim's blood. The toxin will be detected when the sample for investigation is injected into a laboratory mouse which suffers toxicity. The toxin presence therefore is indirectly reflective of the organism's presence. For *Clostridium difficile*, which is an important cause of diarrhea that is antibiotic-associated, a stool sample is obtained, and a filtrate of the same is exposed to laboratory samples of tissue in the test tube. Again, presence of infection is associated with a toxic effect to the tissue.

Genetic Detection

Rather than serology, microbial growth, antigen detection, or determination of bioactivity, the presence of a microbe in a clinical sample can be implied by the finding of genetic material that is specific to the microbe. Living microbes must have a genetic code which is used to specify the replication or production of microbial components. This genetic material may be DNA or RNA. Therefore, the presence of microbial-specific genetic material is indicative of the microbe presence in the context of infection. A detection of genetic material does not require that a live microbe be present (i.e., whether living or not, the genetic material is still present).

Figures 9a and 9b illustrate two general patterns in how genetic detection may take place. Essentially, the genetic material is directly detected, or it is amplified into many copies for detection. The development of these methods is a direct reflection of the many useful tools which have been gained through changes in the field of molecular biology. These particular tools are capable of detecting minute quantities of the microbe and are indeed revolutionary. There are now many different ways in which the genetic material of a microbe could be amplified to facilitate its detection from clinical samples.

Overall, the specific choice of diagnostic method depends on the agent, the available technology, and proof of its validity, as well as the course of the illness.

88

Figures 9 a and b. Methods for genetic detection of microbes in clinical specimens.

a. *Direct probe technology.* In this example, the double-stranded DNA from a bacterium in a given clinical sample is opened into two single strands. After separation, a laboratory derived and labelled short complementary DNA sequence is added which will recognize an area of bacterial DNA. The amount of label measured (e.g., radiolabel or enzyme label) is reflective of the amount of bacterial DNA that was present in the sample.

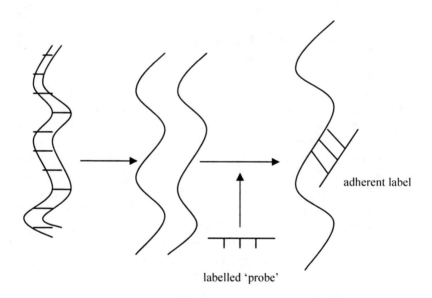

adherent label

labelled 'probe'

b. Genetic amplification. The small amount of microbial DNA or RNA in a clinical sample is reproduced an exponential number of times so that the net result is a large amount of genetic material which can more easily be detected by one of several methods. This particular version is called the **polymerase chain reaction** (PCR). In the example, after the double strand of DNA is dissociated, a short sequence called the primer is added which recognizes a specific region and which serves to signal the reproduction of the strand. The cyclical reproduction of these DNA strands represents the so-called chain reaction.

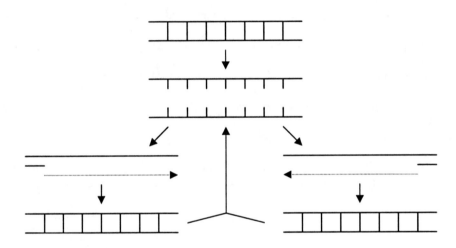

Food For Thought

1. From the time a test is requested by a physician for an ill patient, what problems may arise that could prevent the test result from being a valid one?
2. Define limitations for culture diagnosis of infectious diseases.
3. Define limitations for serological diagnosis of infectious diseases.
4. A critically ill 60 yr. patient is admitted to hospital with severe pneumonia. The patient has been previously well, and there are no risk factors for opportunistic infections. Being liberal with your possibilities, what non-specific and microbe-specific diagnostic measures might be used to establish the diagnosis of infection?

Supplemental Reading

Cimolai N – ed. *Laboratory Diagnosis of Bacterial Infections*. New York, NY:Marcel Dekker, Inc., 2001.
- advanced reading in diagnostic bacteriology and a reference source

de la Maza LM, Pezzlo MJ, Baron EJ. *Color Atlas of Diagnostic Microbiology*. St. Louis, MO:Mosby-Year Book, Inc., 1997.
- advanced but plenty of bright visuals to tease the eye and mind

Forbes BA, Sahm DF, Weissfeld AS. *Bailey and Scott's Diagnostic Microbiology*. 12th Edn. 2007.
- provides good introductions and is sufficiently detailed for the enthusiast

Jerome KR. – ed. *Lennette's Laboratory Diagnosis of Viral Infections*. 5th Edition. New York, NY:Informa Healthcare, USA, Inc., 2010.
- advanced reading in diagnostic virology and a reference source

Winn Jr W, Allen S,, Janda W, Koneman E, Schreckenberger P, Woods G. *Koneman's Colour Atlas and Textbook of Diagnostic Microbiology*. 5th Edn. Philadelphia, PA:Lippincott, 2005.
- a well-illustrated and comprehensive primer for the advanced health professional

"Science is built up with facts, as a house is with stones. But a collection of facts is no more a science than a heap of stones is a house."
Jules Henri Poincard
La Science et l'Hypothèse, 1908

V. The Epidemiology of Infection

"**Epidemiology**" is a broad term which refers to the understanding of the factors which relate to the existence and spread of a disease in a patient group. For our purposes here, the epidemiology of infection refers to the understanding of how infection is viewed in a patient population. It reflects on assessment of how common infection is and how it may vary over time. Epidemiology must include a knowledge of the sources for infections and their distribution. It must also concern itself with the issues of spread for infection, recognizing various modes and their likelihood for perpetuating disease. This study will also look at both patient and environmental factors which impede or contribute to the spread of infection. It is only in understanding these many details that we can begin to define ways to contain infection. In general, the latter ways will be aimed towards preventing spread by interrupting the transmission cycles and furthermore reduce the presence of infection in a population so that secondary disease has lesser probability to arise.

In order for a microbe to be acquired, it must exist somewhere; microbes do not spontaneously develop on their own. The sources of microbes are referred to as '**reservoirs**' for infection. They may include the infected patient, the asymptomatic carrier, or a large diversity of living or inanimate things depending on the specific germ of interest. The infected patient will often carry and then shed considerably more infectious microbes than the **asymptomatic carrier**. The microbe will have multiplied considerably during the usual course of infection. For example, during an active cold, millions or more viruses can be shed from the respiratory tract. The asymptomatic carrier is not evidently diseased by the microbe which is being carried. Some of this carriage may include germs which are temporarily or permanently part of the usual bacteria that inhabits areas of the body. Particular viruses (e.g., Epstein-Barr virus, adenovirus, cytomegalovirus) may actively replicate in the body and yet not actively be associated with an illness. Shedding of these replicating viruses into saliva or urine may serve as reservoir for infection.

Reservoirs for infectious agents in nature abound. These may include insects, mammals, water, soil, and many other foci. Quantitation is considerably variable. Human-made products or modifications of the environment can also serve as reservoirs. There are many examples here, but one of the best known includes food and water supplies. Engineering feats are sometimes proven to be medical foes (e.g., humidifiers and air conditioning towers yielding *Legionella*; hot tubs allowing for overgrowth of *Pseudomonas* causing skin irritation; fish farms allowing for overgrowth of *Streptococcus iniae* which can cause aggressive subcutaneous infection). All of these reservoirs may be cyclical in the quantitation of hazardous microbe carried; cycles of increased risk for spread may occur as a consequence of numerous variables whether crowding, climate, or other. Inside a health care facility, especially hospital, many new reservoirs for infection are created if not only because ill patients are cared for. Items such as beds, handrails, thermometers, stethoscopes, among many other items can be temporary reservoirs when they are tainted by contact with germs. Some of these hospital (**nosocomial**) reservoirs can persist for hours to days; others can be sufficiently cleaned with disinfectants or other processes. Whether patient or object as the reservoir in a hospital, one must recognize the incredible dynamic of change - new patients, reused objects, existing patients being more ill, to name a few. It is evident that the potential to acquire infection of some sort is considerable, and it explains why infections are evidently such a common component of every day life.

For the purposes of infection control, patients and health care workers with infection or colonization serve as the major focus for infections in developed countries. Major reservoirs in this context include the gastrointestinal tract, the respiratory tract, and skin. Much attention therefore is given to patients with the latter infections.

How will infection be transmitted from these sources (Table 1)? It must be initially accepted that some infections will be due to the individual's own microbial flora (e.g., bacteria from intestines or skin will infect surgical wounds) (**auto-infection**). **Cross-infections** refer to the acquisition of germ from a reservoir to a new patient. The method for transfer will usually be direct contact with person or object, most commonly by hand. Respiratory spread (airborne) is important for some infections. The distances travelled may be short (e.g., respiratory spread of cold viruses in large cough or sneezing droplets) or far (e.g., chicken pox spread in a classroom). Given that direct hand transmission is most important in clinic or hospital, the potential role for handwashing to break transmission cannot be overly emphasized. For general community purposes, several other modes of transmission achieve greater importance - water ingestion, food consumption, and insect bites.

When the infecting germ is acquired, there will be a lag time between the time of exposure and the appearance of the first symptoms or signs of active infection - we refer to this interval as the **incubation period**. For some infections, the incubation period may be short (hours to a few days), whereas for others, the incubation period may extend into weeks or months (Table 2).

In detailing the epidemiology of infection, several words are commonly used which deserve explanation; for these are often the vocabulary of infection control. In describing frequency (Table 3), the **prevalence** of infection refers to the number of such infections which exist at any one point in time. For example, the number of individuals who are HIV-positive among the denominator of the population base in a given area defines the prevalence of HIV. The **incidence** of an infection defines the number of new episodes which have occurred in a given unit time. For example, for infections with methicillin-resistant *Staphylococcus aureus* (MRSA) which occurred among seventeen inhabitants of a nursing home during a week, the incidence that week of MRSA infection was 4/17

Table 1. Common routes of spread for infection.

A. Direct person-person contact (hands, secretions, other body-body interactions)
  e.g., *Streptococcus pyogenes* and strep throat
  e.g., antibiotic-resistant Gram negative bacilli in a hospital
  e.g., vancomycin-resistant *Enterococcus faecalis*
  e.g., sexually transmitted diseases

B. Respiratory
  e.g., respiratory viruses
  e.g., whooping cough
  e.g., diphtheria

C. Iatrogenic – instrument derived
  e.g., bacterial spores for surgical instruments when not properly decontaminated

D. Food and water
  e.g., gastrointestinal pathogens
  e.g., some parasites
  e.g., typhoid fever
  e.g., brucellosis

E. Insect vectors
  e.g., see Chapter II

Table 2. Examples of incubation periods for infectious diseases.

Very short
- food-borne botulism: minutes to a few hours
- other toxin-associated food poisonings: 1-12 hours

Short
- viral diarrhea: 1-3 days
- viral respiratory infections: 2-3 days
- plague: 2-4 days
- gonorrhea: 2-7 days
- bacterial diarrhea: 1-4 days

Intermediate
- infectious mononucleosis (Epstein-Barr virus): 1-4 weeks
- primary syphilis: 2-4 weeks
- Q fever: 2-3 weeks
- whooping cough: 1-3 weeks
- Hepatitis B: 1-5 months (usually 2-3 months)
- giardiasis: 1-4 weeks

Long
- leprosy: usually 1-5 years
- rabies: usually 4 weeks to 1 year
- Creutzfeldt-Jakob Disease: 1-30 years

Table 3. Frequencies for some global infectious diseases.

Tuberculosis	~10-20 million
Leprosy	~ 5 million
Schistosomiasis	>200 million
Dracunculiasis (guinea worm)	~100,000
Human immunodeficiency virus (HIV)	>50 million
Hepatitis B	~500,000 deaths per year

(approximately 24%). An **outbreak** has occurred when the number of infections over a unit of time has exceeded an anticipated number of infections. The anticipated number will be determined with the knowledge of past experience which has in essence determined the baseline or norm. The determination of what constitutes an excess above the norm is often clear-cut, but at times may be arbitrary. An outbreak of influenza in a school may involve scores of children. Yet, an outbreak may be defined as well by four urinary tract infections with *Serratia marcescens* in a hospital urology ward where there were previously none. Therefore, whereas a large number of infections can be readily identified as an outbreak, a small number of identical infections in a closed environment where none first exist may be termed the same. **Epidemic** is but a synonym for outbreak, although most will use this term when the actual numbers of infected are great. **Pandemic** describes epidemic activity that is very wide-spread. One may have an influenza epidemic which affects a hospital ward, and one may have a pandemic of influenza which is afflicting the world (H1N1 virus epidemic of 2009-2010).

We have previously detailed the variability of microbes which cause infection. Given genetic variability among humans, it is evident how there may be considerable differences for patients, whether of their immune systems, their other body tissues which interact with a microbe, or their non-immune host defences. The permutations of microbial-human interaction are astounding. Modern medicine has achieved wonders, but we must realize that for some patients, medical treatment occurs at the risk of making individuals <u>more</u> susceptible to infection. With the body either acutely or chronically weakened, new categories of microbes are capable of causing infection which would otherwise be exceedingly uncommon to cause illness. The latter microbes lead to **opportunistic infection**. The fungus *Aspergillus fumigatus*, which is common in the environment, will rarely be responsible for infection in the otherwise normal individual, but it is a dreaded pathogen for patients with severe immune compromise. Not only do opportunistic microbes present themselves as a new foe, but the related infections may be both more difficult to diagnose and to treat. Age-related susceptibility is also but one of the number of variables that will affect the epidemiology of a particular infection (Table 4).

Infections which take place in a setting where there are large numbers of patients, where infections are common, and where relative crowding occurs must then certainly be at high risk for spread. Such is the hospital environment and similar large institutional settings. Nosocomial infections particularly include microbes, especially bacteria, which have more resistance to antibiotics than usual. The latter problem is compounded when the most potent of antibiotics are used which then furthers the potential for increasing resistance. A **nosocomial infection** occurs when the infection has not been present at the time of hospital admission. Usually such an infection will occur at earliest approximately two days after admission. In contrast, a **community-acquired infection** is either

Table 4. Factors which may affect the epidemiology of infectious diseases.

Age	History of sexual activity
Anatomic defects	Illicit drug use
Antibiotic use	Immune compromise
Clinical status	Nutritional status
Dose of pathogen	Presence of other infections
Duration of exposure	Receipt of blood products
Employment	Socioeconomic status
Exposure in a crowded environment	Travel
Exposure in a hospital	Underlying illness
Exposure to a disease vector	Vaccination
Food exposure	Virulence of the microbe
Genetics	Water exposure
Geography	

incubating or actively present on initial patient contact.

There are many potential body sites for infection, and an infection at any of these sites may be apparent through a spectrum of disease manifestations. The following infections or manifestations are among the most common:

Fever
Rash and other direct skin infections
Upper Respiratory Tract Infections (includes external ear and eye)
Lower Respiratory Infections
Urinary Tract Infections
Gastrointestinal Tract Infections
Wound Infections
Genital and Reproductive Infections
Blood-Borne Infections
Central Nervous System Infections
Bone and Joint Infections

Life is only as complicated as we make it. This phrase is evermore so applicable to infections and their control.

Food For Thought

1. What incubation periods are there for the following infections;
      - chicken pox?
      - measles (rubeola)?
      - tuberculosis?
2. How extensively distributed are *Legionella* species in the environment?
3. Can you recall citations of infectious epidemics that have been cited in the news over the last year?
4. What infections can be transmitted from water sources?

Supplemental Reading

Aguirre AA, Tabor GM. Global factors driving emerging infectious diseases. *Ann NY Acad Sci* Vol. 1149:pages 1-3 (2008).
- how the world around us may have impact on the infections we suffer

Cimolai N. MRSA and the environment: implications for comprehensive control measures. *Eur J Clin Microbiol Infect Dis* Vol. 27:pages 481-493 (2008).
- a good example of the environmental role for potential transmission of a very topical pathogen: methicillin-resistant *Staphylococcus aureus*

Cliver DO, Potter M, Riemann HP. *Foodborne Infections and Intoxications*. 3rd Edition. Waltham, MA:Academic Press/Elsevier, 2005.
- will you ever eat again?

Collins CH, Aw TC, Grange JM. *Microbial Diseases of Occupation, Sports, and Recreations*. Boston, MA:Butterworth-Heinimann, 1997.
- specific interests for the enthusiast

Giesecke J. *Modern Infectious Disease Epidemiology*. 2nd Edition. New York, NY:Oxford University Press, 2002.
- a good overview

Lafferty KD. The ecology of climate change and infectious diseases. *Ecology* Vol. 90:pages 888-901 (2009).
- a role for global environmental changes

Webber R. *Communicable Disease Epidemiology and Control: A Global Perspective*. 3rd Edition. Oxford, UK:CAB International, 2009.
- a nicely illustrated primer with plenty of detail for the health care professional

"What's in a name? That which we call a rose
By any other name would smell as sweet."
William Shakespeare
Romeo and Juliet II, ii, 43
(Note: one author's recitation to the other co-author)

VI. What's In a Name?

Change must be appreciated for what it is worth. Can anyone that has participated in health care deny the phenomenal changes of the last few decades? In the microbiology arena, we have witnessed changing concepts, new pathogens, newly understood infectious diseases and their evolution, as well as changes in the actual terminology of microbial names. The area of infection control has had its own changes, especially in regards to our fundamental descriptions of how we carry on with our business. Infection control has a long history as we have detailed in the first chapter. Many of the major impediments for infection control were consolidated in decades past. Yet, contemporary times have led to some confusion if not only because of how we have used different terms to describe our practice. If there is one driving force that has especially led to revisionary pathways, it is the recognition of HIV and the AIDS era. Thereafter, the SARS epidemics and H1N1 influenza pandemic of recent have reinforced the same.

Prior to the 1980s, descriptions of infection and the methods for their containment (**quarantine**) were in place. General approaches for the management of patients with common respiratory infections and gastroenteritis, for example, were utilized. As well, a general sense of precaution with the emphasis on handwashing in addition to category-specific precautions was accepted. **Category-specific precautions** were designed to apply infection control to clusters of similar infections. In the area of blood-borne pathogens, however, it was essentially hepatitis B that was thought to be of peril. Patients so infected were placed on **Blood and Body Fluid Precautions** openly with the adoption of thinking that contact with these body substances was predominantly associated with transmission. Special precautions were maintained for contact with the patient's blood or deep fluids especially when blood-tinged. Essentially, patients with known hepatitis B carrier status or those with acute hepatitis were so managed, but little emphasis was placed on the unknown (i.e., the asymptomatic carrier of hepatitis B that was undiagnosed). The latter lack of concern was perhaps influenced by the then putative low frequencies of chronic hepatitis B carriage in some geographical areas. Perhaps the deficit might have seemed inappropriate in retrospect, but it was also a time when preventative techniques were poor (e.g., no available hepatitis B vaccine). The advent of HIV and AIDS, and then consolidated with the arrival of hepatitis C, triggered an interest in the unknown. Despite now an apparent small frequency of HIV-infected patients, the consequences of infection acquisition were great. Concern for unrecognized infection seemed sensible. The issue of confidentiality also had its own impact. Although the understanding of Blood and Body Fluids Precautions could be applied to a chronic carrier of hepatitis B openly, general knowledge of HIV status carried with it many more concerns and controversies with respect to confidentiality. Accordingly, health care workers were recognized to require precautions for general purposes but to also ensure the maintenance of confidentiality. These concerns were seemingly integral to the development of **Universal Precautions** in which due care was to be given for contact with all human specimens.

To some, the theme of Universal Precautions was but a supplement to existing practice. In addition to various categories of precaution (see next Chapter) which had been adopted for many years, a special sense of urgency was established to ensure that all body substances would be treated with respect, even when an infection diagnosis was not established. From the patient perspective, equal treatment and privacy regardless of the diagnosis seemed acceptable. At least the term and narrow view of Blood and Body Precautions was lost. Most health care centres then embraced the concept of Universal Precautions quickly; some continue to subscribe to such guidelines as originally conceived.

Others, however, believed that Universal Precautions, in its detailed description, focused overly on the issue of maintaining concern for body substances that were overtly tainted with blood. For example, urine, stool, and breast milk that were not evidently blood-tainted might be exempted from Universal Precautions. Still others evolved a sense of complacency in that, whereas Universal Precautions would apply to all patients, perhaps Universal Precautions might apply to all infections. The latter misconception required ongoing effort to remind individuals of the original concepts.

With concern that Universal Precautions was perhaps overly restrictive by the initial proposals that concern be given to substances which had obvious or likely blood contamination, the term **Body Substance Precautions** arose. Here, all body substances were deemed to carry risk whether or not blood was evident. Clearly, these concerns were scientifically valid since microscopic contamination with blood, which would therefore imply tainting with blood-borne pathogens, might not be visualized, and since furthermore, some body substances might harbor these pathogens without ever having been blood-tainted (e.g., semen). Nevertheless, whereas the latter was indeed credible, most health care workers had already become familiar with the Universal Precautions terminology and continued to use the same while proceeding to encompass the valid concerns of Body Substance Precautions. We must be consistent in recognizing that on most practical bases, these infection control approaches are essentially synonymous.

Enter **Standard Precautions**. Perhaps the Universal Precautions designation did carry with it a misunderstanding of uniformity related to all infections, rather than all patients, even if this was not the intent. The term Standard Precautions implies a consistency of minimum standard which should be applied to all patients. Whether obviously seeded with blood or not, all body substances have a potential to carry infectious agents and must therefore be considered for having the potential to infect the health care worker. Whereas certain substances are of greater risk (e.g., bloody tissues versus visually untainted urine), the health care worker has the obligation to assess risk in a given situation and behave accordingly. Just as thought may be given to ascertain that specific items may be recognized to carry varying degrees of risk, the health care worker must equally consider methods of prevention. Standard Precautions then refers to the general methods by which acquisition of infection is reduced, and as such, they are applicable to all patients one may encounter, whether in hospital or not and whether evidently infected or not. This basic minimum is then the foundation upon which more category-specific precautions are added when appropriate according to the specific infection being encountered. These terminologies might be more likely applied in medical institutions, but their intent is applicable to the transmission of infection in any venue.

What's in a name?

Food For Thought

1. In what body fluids and secretions has the human immunodeficiency virus (HIV) been found?
2. Define Standard Precautions.
3. A pressure blister on the foot of a 17 year old female athlete has ruptured. What infectious hazards are there for this person's trainer?

Supplemental Reading
(experience using medical literature peer-reviewed journals for the ultimate in brain-storming)

Consider the following references as being representative of current thought from the last

102

decade:

Academy of Pediatrics. Infection control in physicians' offices. *Pediatrics* Vol. 105: pages 1361-1369 (2000).
- a view of how standard precautions would be applied in the ambulatory area

Cutter J, Gammon J. Review of standard precautions and sharps management in the community. *British Journal of Nursing* Vol. 12: pages 54-60 (2007).
- further views on ambulatory infection prevention

Gammon J, Morgan-Samuel H, Gould D. A review of the evidence for suboptimal compliance of healthcare practitioners to standard/universal infection control precautions. *Journal of Clinical Nursing* Vol. 17: pages 157-167 (2008).
- how a good idea translates (or does not) into healthcare practice

Molinari JA. Infection control: its evolution to the current standard precautions. *Journal of the American Dental Association.* Vol. 134: pages 569-574 (2003).
- although focused on dentistry, this review has its practical and universal merits

Consider the following references for a look into the past and the way in which changing terminologies were applied:

West KH, Cohen ML. Standard precautions – a new approach to reducing infection in the hospital setting. *Journal of Intravenous Nursing* Vol. 20 (Supplement 6): pages 7-10 (1997).
- standard precautions was being introduced in North America over the preceding year

Hopkins CC. Implementation of universal blood and body fluid precautions. *Infectious Disease Clinics of North America* Vol. 3: pages 747-762 (1989).
- looking at things historically

Hughes JM. Universal precautions: CDC perspective. *Occupational Medicine* Vol. 4 (Supplement): pages 13-20 (1989).
- looking at things historically

Duncan IB, Batchelor C. Assessment of the effectiveness of body substance precautions as the infection control system of a large teaching hospital. *American Journal of Infection Control* Vol. 21: pages 302-309 (1993).
- a description of practical experience

Gerberding JL, Lewis FR Jr., Schecter WP. Are universal precautions realistic? *Surgical Clinics of North America.* Vol. 75: pages 1091-1104 (1995).
- dive head first into the controversy as it existed then

"He that hath clean hands, and a pure heart."
Psalms 24:1-4

VII. Methods of Prevention and Quarantine

Managing Behaviour

The basic elements of effective infection control are seemingly elementary when viewed as line items in a written protocol. How much more fundamental can a technique be than handwashing? Yet, constant reminders are required to ensure the implementation of simple principles. These simple principles are cause for discussion, debate, disharmony at times, and doubt. It is no wonder that they maybe the basis for a book!

As science must be a pillar of good medicine, so too is it a foundation for good infection control. Yet, whereas the infections may be new, complex, or changing, the basic infection control practices have changed very little. A scientific knowledge will be used in most if not all decisions or practices of infection control, but one can easily down-play the quantity. We must admit that on a proportionate basis, infection control is 95% behavior modification and 5% science.

Many practices are generally carried out in contexts where most have received an advanced education of some form. It would seem that the adoption of infection control should be more easily accomplished. So little truth is there in the latter however. Knowledge is important, but it does not in itself modify attitude and complacency. Many see infection control as a bureaucratic regime - punitive and unbending. Little is it recognized that the actual implementation of safe infection control is a component of life for all us, no matter what area the health care worker emphasizes. In times lacking infections, infection control is a burden. In times of incident, those who previously declined participation are either nowhere to be seen or are friendly allies. The basic standards should be the eternal norm.

Risk Management or Risk Reduction?

It would be desirable to prevent the occurrence and then secondary transmission of all infections, but from a practical perspective, this may never be possible. Instead, a reasonable reduction of either could be accepted depending on the circumstances. Infection control practices will never be able to prevent the transmission of all infections. Therefore, the practice of infection control must identify and thereafter implement appropriate patterns of behavior in order to minimize disease and to ensure that the outcomes are generally acceptable to medical and lay constituencies.

The theme of **risk management** is common to medicine as it is in many other venues. Essentially, risk management refers to the efforts which work towards the goal of reducing unplanned or unexpected events for an individual organization. In health care, risk management will be applicable to both patient and health care worker. It requires judgments to be made about the magnitude of health risk as well as economic, health, and social consequences of taking particular precautions to reduce the exposure and hence risk.

Risk management must by definition include **risk assessment**, and risk assessment in turn includes four basic components. We know that infectious agents are capable of leading to adverse health impact; the acknowledgment of infectious agents represents an **identification of hazard**. In the process of measuring the intensity, duration, and frequency of exposures to the microbe, we provide an **exposure measurement**. Defining the relationship between exposure and the frequency of an adverse event occurring provides a **dose-response assessment**. The latter three judgments will then culminate in **risk characterization** which estimates the chances of an adverse event occurring under various conditions, or context, of the exposure.

The 'scales' of infection control are similar to those of the 'scales' of justice; perhaps all who practice infection control should have been born under the zodiac sign of Libra! Infection control has a strong sense of justice and must carefully weigh opposing concerns. Through science and diplomacy, infection control seeks balance. It must be diplomatic, precise, intelligent, and socially understanding. It must exercise reason and leadership. In the end, the cost of prevention must have been worth the cost of cure.

Essential Ingredients

Having considered the possible modes of acquiring microbes (Chapter V), there are obviously a finite number of ways in which such acquisition can be prevented. Total abstinence from interaction with anything or anyone is sure to prevent transmission, but it is at the same time an unrealistic expectation. Nevertheless, the use of a totally inanimate and "sterile" environment for children with major inborn immune deficiencies ("Bubble Babies") proved that this concept was not entirely without promise. Conversely, the practical approach to infection control relies on the employment of at least seven essential and basic ingredients. Use of these may occur simply or in various combinations: (a) handwashing, (b) gloving, (c) face/mucous membrane protection, (d) gowning, (e) decontamination, (f) ventilation, and (g) inanition.

Handwashing

Handwashing is said by some to be the most important single component of good infection control practice. The skin is a relatively good anatomic barrier to microbes entering the body, but nevertheless it is a site where bacteria normally reside. The quantity of usual bacteria on the skin is quite variable, but most such bacteria are generally non-pathogenic. On some occasions, bacteria with greater virulence potential can be found on the skin including those that originate in the nose or mouth, the gastrointestinal tract, the genitourinary tract, and the environment. The sources for these bacteria may be the individual or other individuals. Although bacteria from another individual are most likely to be acquired during direct contact, it is also possible that the microbes have been temporarily transferred to an inanimate object which then allows for some transient survival until that time that they are contacted by hands once more. Most bacteria from other anatomic sites tend to be only transiently carried on the hands, but a few (e.g., *S. aureus*, enterococci) can become resident. The folds and fingernails further add to the potential for bacteria to remain. The degree of contamination of skin will depend on the initial quantity of contamination as well as the number and intensity of repeat contacts thereafter. For example, the caregiver who is required to attend to incontinent bed-ridden elderly patients or the individual who changes toddler diapers is quite likely to have hands soiled with fecal-source bacteria. Overall, there is ample opportunity for the hands of the health care worker to become soiled with pathogenic bacteria, and it only requires the presence of very few viable pathogenic bacteria to colonize and then infect the subsequent recipient of the next hand contact. In many circumstances, the value of handwashing has been re-affirmed in scientific studies, thus validating what might seem intuitive to many.

What constitutes good handwashing? Many have sought to define good handwashing practice by detailing technique, length of work, and nature of the handwash product. Such definitions may serve as a standard, but it is evident that the exact technique must be warranted by the need or context. There is both a mechanical and an antimicrobial component to good handwashing. The mechanical component consists of the running water, the assurance that the decontaminating effect includes all of the hand surface, and the rubbing manoeuvers. The antimicrobial component includes the actual inhibitory or microbial-killing (**germicidal**) properties of the soap or chemical as well as its potential ability to provide some form of detergent-like action. General purpose soap is usually adequate for handwashing. In the washing of hands, a detergent effect may be desirable to allow for hand soilage to be freed from the skin; a detergent agent in itself will also have some potential antibacterial properties by way largely of destabilizing the bacterial surface and limiting membrane (Figure 1). Other handwashing agents may contain variable chemicals that have antibacterial properties through several mechanisms (see Chapter VIII)(e.g., the 'surgical scrub' makes use of prolonged washing with an antiseptic). These

Figure 1. The effect of a detergent to disrupt the fatty bilayer of a bacterial cell membrane.

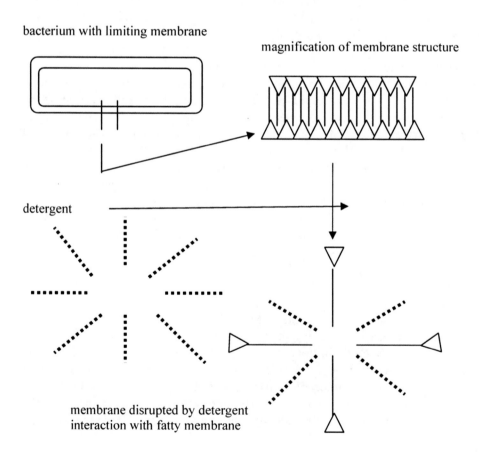

bacterium with limiting membrane

magnification of membrane structure

detergent

membrane disrupted by detergent interaction with fatty membrane

agents often differ in their ability to neutralize different bacteria and in the speed at which such antagonism occurs. It is critical, however, to accept the fact that handwashing agents are not absolute or anywhere near absolute in their ability to rid the hands of germs. The relative antibacterial effect is dependent on the initial microbial load. If the germ load is high and the ability of the antimicrobial to neutralize is limited to a certain quantitation over time, it is quite possible that microbes, even pathogenic ones, may continue to be present even when the majority is eradicated. In a given period of time, which may measure many minutes to several hours, the original quantity of microbial burden may be restored due to growth. If the agent simply inhibits rather than kills the germ, growth will also continue after a recovery period which is variable and is dependent on the specific activity of the given agent. For example, if one were to wash hands and then use gloves for an extended period of time thereafter (e.g., long surgical procedure), the survival of a few germs from handwashing would then translate into a multitude of germs after many hours when microbial growth returns, especially in the heat and moisture of the gloves. The antimicrobial agent will not be active at sites where it cannot penetrate the microbial residence. Thus, whereas handwashing remains an important essential ingredient in infection control practice, it is not absolute in its ability to achieve control. Even good handwashing may leave a margin of error for further communicability, and even more so, the best handwashing technique or antibacterial agent may fail when hands become contaminated once again from re-contact.

Whereas it is clear that the hands should be washed after obvious contamination, it is ideal that handwashing should be performed after each unique patient encounter. Table 1 details some sensible opportune occasions for handwashing. It may even be prudent to handwash between procedures for the same patient depending on context. It is the potential burden of such activity, however, that in reality modifies the ideal to some acceptable (in the caregivers' eyes) compromise. When infection control procedures are seemingly minimal, this balance is tipped towards convenience; when problems are evident, it becomes easier for caregivers to comply. It is human nature to shun less desirable activity.

In order to achieve adequate washing, there must be reasonable provision for a safe and proximal water source. Sinks need to be close to patient care areas. Both health care workers and patients/families/supportive individuals must have ready access. Where hands are washed and dried with paper towels at the care site, it is wise to use the paper hand drying towel to turn off the tap. There are now new technologies which distribute both soap and water using touchless systems, and such a trend approaches the ideal.

The last decade has seen the promulgation of alcohol hand rubs (liguid,

Table 1. Key opportunities for handwashing.

> before and after patient contact

> certainly after contact with secretions, excretions, wounds, body fluids, and blood

> upon arriving from outside of a healthcare facility

> upon leaving a healthcare facility

> after removing gloves and other protective apparel

> before and after patient procedures

> after removal of gloves

> to follow personal hygiene needs (e.g., fecal, urinary)

> prior to food handling and after meals

gel, and others) which have been touted to replace handwashing in areas where water supply is most cumbersome. Such drying hand rubs have been proven to show antibacterial efficacy but should not entirely replace good regular handwashing.

Gloving

The use of **gloves** in intended to provide a physical barrier in addition to skin, and the use must be gauged against anticipated risk during patient contact. For example, gloves are generally worn when the caregiver is about to touch infected sites or contaminated items, mucous membranes, blood, body fluids, and body secretions. The routine changing of diapers is usually exempt with the exception of handling patients with presumed infectious enteritides. Nevertheless, gloving is not an absolute protective barrier, and handwashing should always follow the removal of gloves. Gloves should not be re-used, and they should be changed between patient contacts. Even the best of gloves may be susceptible to minor perforations; even gloves newly from the manufacturer may have microperforations. Gloves cannot be considered an absolute substitute for handwashing!

Non-sterile gloves can be used for many routine patient-related processes where barrier protection for the heathcare worker is important. Sterile gloves are more critical when the patient needs to be protected during their treatment.

The use of gloves has taken a further step in the era of greater concern over blood-borne pathogens. Gloves add an extra measure of prevention when needle-stick injuries occur. Again, they are not absolute in this regard, but the need for a sharp to pass through the glove serves to factor in a barrier which removes some of the infectious fluid. It was believed at one time that the risk of needle-stick exposure was the same with or without gloves; this is no longer the case. Hence, it is prudent to wear gloves during procedures which provide risk for skin puncture (e.g., venipuncture).

Just as we are realizing the benefits of wearing gloves, we must also be cognizant of the hazards to a few from latex exposure. Such hazard is usually a form of allergy which may range from simple contact dermatitis to more complex allergic phenomena. There are now non-latex variations which are suitable. These include vinyl and nitrile gloves.

Face/Mucous Membrane Exposure (goggles, masks, shields)

The use of **masks** in order to promote surgical asepsis has a long history, but the primary intention here is simply to prevent the contamination of the operative site by usual oral bacteria from the operator. In this regard, there is likely to be some benefit, but many have challenged the science of mask use. For patients that have a low risk for infection after a procedure (e.g., suture of a skin wound in an out-patient setting), it is probable that masks have little to do with further risk reduction. For those patients who have much to lose from an infection which complicates an advanced procedure (e.g., open hip surgery), even a perceived reduction in risk, albeit small, may be welcome. In part, masking in a particular context, (e.g., anaesthetist in an operating room) can be a reminder of the appropriate behaviour overall that is conducive to the prevention of infection. Many analyses have been made of the airflow that escapes the edge of masks and of the efficiency of mask materials to exclude or trap particles, and there is no routinely-used mask that is perfect. Again, it must be understood that the intent is risk reduction of an acceptable degree.

Masks may also be used for preventing infection among health care workers. Some examples of illnesses among patients that may warrant the use of masks includes tuberculosis, virus respiratory infections, and acute meningococcal infection. The likelihood of acquiring respiratory-borne infections is proportional to the intensity of infection in the patient, length of time of patient exposure, and proximity to the patient. The potential severity of tuberculosis along with the development of drug-resistant tuberculosis has prompted the use of masks with greater efficiency and tighter fit at least for this specific example. In the last decade, concerns for such efficacy in the medical setting came forward largely with the heightened awareness that arose over SARS and influenza epidemics. Masks with proven high efficiency were then promoted and standardized. For example, the N95 designation proposal for mask-respirators by the U.S. National Institute for Occupational Safety and Health establishes a standard whereby the apparatus is capable of excluding particles with a 95% efficiency for 0.3 microns when the operator has been 'fit-tested' for the given make and model. Many have adopted the latter. Keep in mind that <u>most</u> masks that are used in healthcare do <u>not</u> meet such stringent requirements.

It goes without saying that masks should be replaced between patients when there is good reason to believe that the mask can become soiled. One may require a mask change if it is to be used for prolonged periods.

For those who may doubt the validity of masks in the above settings, the role of masks in preventing mucosal soilage with patient blood and other body fluids is a solid counter-argument. The mucous membranes of the eye and mouth may represent relatively inefficient sites for infection with blood-borne viral agents, but they are nevertheless opportune sites. The use of goggles, face shields, and safety glasses are extensions of such preventative potential.

There may also be a role for masking patients when patient transport is required and respiratory droplets pose a great hazard.

Gowning

Gowning mainly serves to protect the health care worker's garments from becoming soiled. Although touted also as a potential mechanism for reducing person-to-person transmission, there is little in the way of concrete evidence to support the latter. In general, there has been a trend to 'de-gowning' especially in the context of nurseries. Gowning may have some role as a reminder to health care workers about overall hygienic needs and standards; the benefits of this approach may greatly outweigh the resources that are needed for gowning.

Gowns tend to be used for high risk procedures or when soiling is likely. Ideally, gowns should be impermeable for fluids. They should only be used for single procedures. The reuse of gowns between patients may serve as a hazard.

When gowns are used upon entry to a patient care area, they should be removed as the healthcare worker exits that same area.

Decontamination

The principles are largely discussed in the next chapter, but essentially it encompasses those methods, procedures, or agents which are used to markedly reduce or totally eliminate the presence of infectious microbes. Three commonly-used words aptly describe what may be accomplished. **Sterilization** assumes that any microbe (living or dormant) will be eliminated. The harsh conditions of heat or chemical necessitate that utilization will be applicable only to inanimate objects. **Disinfection** will also attempt to nullify harmful microbes but not in an absolute sense. For example, a household disinfectant may adequately reduce the risk of acquiring infectious bacteria which have contaminated a counter-top but will not have necessarily eliminated all germs. This term is also generally applied to processes for inanimate objects. An **antiseptic** reduces infection-causing microbes at the body site where they are present (e.g., oral antiseptics such as mouthwashes temporarily decrease counts of oral bacteria). The extent of decontamination that may be preferable is dictated by the given context and is mainly a function of the risk reduction that is deemed acceptable.

Ventilation

There are many examples of infection where the transmission of infection has little if not anything to do with aerosolization. Thus, the **ventilation** of an isolation room for infection control may seemingly be extra-ordinary. To the contrary, there are several examples when particular ventilation standards are critical. For example, the rates of air exchange in operating rooms are specified by recommendations that ensure clean air during the operative procedure, whereby filtered air is exhausted after it passes through the room. Although the frequencies of infection after clean surgery are most often small, many studies of air flow in operative suites and subsequent infection indicate an incremental benefit for prevention of rare but serious infections after complicated surgery. In addition, infections such as chickenpox and tuberculosis are commonly transmitted by aerosols, and thus the prevention of such infections benefits from the use of rooms which have negative pressure ventilation (the room is negative pressure relative to the corridor and draws air in) where room air is exhausted to the outdoors. For respiratory virus infections due to common agents such cold viruses (e.g., rhinoviruses, coronaviruses, influenza, and respiratory syncytial virus), most spread is likely to occur by direct person-person contact but may also occur by large particle aerosols or droplets. The latter are more likely to allow for transmission when individuals are close to the index patient. The role of negative pressure ventilation is disputable in the latter situation. There is also some debate regarding the role of negative pressure ventilation in the prevention of spread for MRSA which may colonize skin. Positive pressure ventilation (air filtered and forced through the room with exhaust to the corridor) is rarely used in the context where the patient requires protection (e.g., critical stages in bone marrow transplantation when patients have intense immunosuppression and susceptibility to infection).

Inanition

If ingestion of microbes via water and food acts as a mechanism for transmission, it is only natural that the interruption of such ingestion will prevent food-borne illnesses. This interruption may not necessarily represent the actual prevention of ingestion altogether but rather will most often be accomplished by proper treatment (e.g., cooking, e.g., preventing contamination) of the water or food. Whereas this method of prevention may not be particularly applicable to most patients in hospital, it represents a critical strategy in the general community. There may be rare circumstances (e.g., during the peak immunosuppression of bone marrow transplantation) when only cooked food may be fed to a patient in order to reduce exposure to environmental organisms such as fungi.

Isolation Techniques

Isolation techniques, whether in hospital, ambulatory settings, or in the community, are systems by which the essential ingredients are united to achieve prevention. These techniques are sometimes referred to as **categories of isolation**. They apply mainly to the quarantine of patients in health care institutions, especially hospitals, but some can also be at times extended to other situations. As indicated in Chapter VI, Standard Precautions implies the application of particular standards to all patient contacts. Isolation techniques are refinements achieved by addenda to these basic principles, and they assist with the handling of common or specific needs. These isolation techniques may be referred to by some authorities as **'transmission-based'** since they are named according to clusters of infections that have particular forms of spread. The need for quarantine is often indicated by the term **'Isolation'**, and hence this word is used in several of these techniques. Whereas some of these categories are so designated by the descriptions to follow, there are insititutions that use synonyms which are held steadfastly by them. The specific title may not be so much important as long as health care workers fully appreciate the intent and eventually activate safe practices. The intent may be absolute prevention or risk reduction depending on the circumstances. Signs which indicate that the patient is quarantined under certain precautions should be posted and easily identified.

These should outline the technique in lay terms. All visitors who are new to the patient's room should report initially to the supervisory health care workers.

For the purpose of being informative, we chose to identify five major isolation techniques which include: Contact Isolation, Enteric Isolation, Respiratory Isolation, Strict Isolation, and Protective Isolation. Some choose to use the term '**Precautions**' rather than 'Isolation' (e.g., Respiratory Precautions rather than Respiratory Isolation). Furthermore, others may rely on slightly different terminologies to use in every day practice. For example, '**Transmission-Based Precautions**', as an overview term, has been adopted by many, emanating from authorities in the U.S. Rather than the categories of isolation that we detail herein, the Transmission-Based Precautions are divided into three main approaches: Contact Precautions, Droplet Precautions, and Airborne Precautions. Yet other institutions worldwide have adopted alternate labels. At the end of the day, it is not the title that is important but rather the content and intent of any such isolation technique that matters. It should not practically speaking be difficult for healthcare workers to adapt to these varying names - again, the posting of key facets for implementation for a given patient upon entry into the room will smoothe out any such problem.

There are occasions when combinations of isolation techniques may be used for a given patient. There may also be occasions when multiple patients are cared for in a common area; all quarantined for the same concern and using the same isolation technique (e.g., three young children all admitted to the same ward and who suffer from parainfluenza 3 virus infection). When patients first arrive and a form of isolation is invoked, a more overreaching technique may be initially chosen, then to be modified to a more refined precaution once the diagnosis is established. Discontinuation of any quarantine may then depend on the completion of a predetermined typical infectious period or after the determination that infection has been terminated as deemed by laboratory methods.

Most important, however, is that isolation techniques can only be highly efficient when the physical lay-out and resources required are reliably provided. Certainly, they can only be effectively implemented when both caregivers and the cared-for buy in.

Contact Isolation

This technique has also been referred to as Barrier Isolation or Drainage and Skin Precautions. The intent is to prevent the transmission of infections for which the major if not only mechanism for spread is direct contact. Examples of such infections might include post-surgical wound infection, skin infections after trauma otherwise, impetigo, and scabies. In the current era where antibiotic-resistant bacteria may colonize a patient, such a technique will be employed in order to minimize spread. In this scenario, transmission may occur via direct contact with the infection or indirectly when material from the infected site contaminates inanimate objects.

The stringency by which this technique is applied will be a function of the specific pathogen or type of infection. For example, a wound that is profusely draining pus or a *S. pyogenes*-associated necrotizing fasciitis would be treated more cautiously than a nearly healed post-appendectomy scar that may have some coliform bacteria. If the site of infection is focal, it may be amenable to cover with a dressing that in itself reduces the risk for spread of infection. Placement of the patient in a single room may be helpful but is not obligatory.

Gloves are worn when handling the patient, especially the wound itself. Regardless, a handwashing station should be accessible. A gown for the health care worker is also recommended but only when there is patient contact. The mere entry and exit from a room is not sufficient to warrant gloves or gown when there is no patient contact. Patients with different reasons for Contact Isolation may be cared for in the same room, but health care workers will be required to change gloves and gown between patients. A mask may be advocated when the wound is subject to dressing changes or irrigation.

Enteric Isolation

Enteric Isolation is applied to prevent the spread of infections that are most likely to be spread by the fecal-oral mode of contamination. Thus, these patients most commonly will have gastrointestinal infections with viruses or bacteria (e.g., rotavirus, enteric adenovirus, *Salmonella*). Direct or indirect contact with contaminated fecal material may allow for the health care worker to autoinfect when the mouth is touched by the contaminated hand. In many respects, this technique is but a slight variation of Contact Isolation, and this is why some have elected to combine Contact Isolation and Enteric Isolation into one brand (e.g., Contact Precautions as per Transmission-Based Precautions).

The patient will often be placed in a single room, but it is possible to have patients with different enteric pathogens in the same room as long as they can be sufficiently segregated and given that toilet facilities are not shared. Likewise, a patient in Enteric Isolation may be maintained in a room with other patients if the precautions and segregation can be enforced. Patients who have an enteric infection but are continent pose less of a risk, but they should be reminded of the need to wash their hands as well as their restriction from food handling and preparation while in the health care institution. Gloves should be worn when there is opportunity that contact may be had with infected excreta or secretions (e.g., vomitus). Masks are not usually necessary. Infected excreta may be discarded via the regular outlets (e.g., toilet). Gowns should be worn when there is direct patient contact or when it is anticipated that soilage with excreta or contaminated objects is a real possibility. Handwashing facilities should be practically accessible.

Respiratory Isolation

Although germs which are associated with respiratory spread via breathing, sneezing, and coughing may yet be transmitted between patients by direct contact, there are additional precautions which prevent the airborne spread. Essentially the intent is to prevent the contact between aerosolized germs and the health care worker or visitors' respiratory tract where these infections are initiated.

In the best case scenario, patients are quarantined in single rooms which have been designed with negative pressure ventilation and door closure. A mask is worn to prevent aerosol contact. Gloves are worn when there is a need to handle the patient, respiratory secretions, or objects in the vicinity which have a high probability for contamination. The use of gowns is recommended, although the relative contribution may be debated. If patients under this quarantine are to leave their room for diagnostic and treatment measures, they should wear a mask.

Not all infections which are potentially transmitted by aerosols are as easily spread; some are more likely to be transmitted by large particle aerosols rather than small ones. For example, chickenpox can be transmitted efficiently through small aerosols that may extend over a modest-length hallway. In contrast, most transmissions of respiratory syncytial virus in an institutional setting occur by direct contact or via large particle aerosol (over a few feet). Given the manner in which such large particles (virus and respiratory secretions sent by coughing, etc.) settle in air, they are likely to be acquired with very close contact. As the distance increases between caregiver and patient, the risk of spread decreases proportionately. Indeed, some argue whether negative pressure ventilation is of much value, if at all required (e.g., the Droplet Precautions mode from Transmission-Based Precautions does not promote special air handling and ventilation). The resources available in an institution may strongly dictate what may be implemented in this regard, but new building designs can take such needs into consideration.

The quarantine for tuberculosis is an extension of Respiratory Isolation, but a modification for including more efficient masks has been suggested by some. In an era where drug-resistant tuberculosis is a reality in some centres, more vigilance is exercised in preventing aerosol spread – higher efficiency and tighter-fitting masks will be used (e.g., fit-tested N95) (In Transmission-Based Precautions, examples such as measles virus, chickenpox virus, tuberculosis, and SARS-CoV attract Airborne Precautions).

Strict Isolation

This technique is essentially an extension of respiratory isolation. It reflects an extreme position in preventing infection that may be regarded as highly communicable or highly lethal. Patients are cared for in a single room that has **negative pressure ventilation**. All entrants wear mask and gown; gloves are included when there is patient contact.

This form of isolation may be applied to active chickenpox. Some also prefer to use this method for containment of MRSA especially when the facility has the physical resources, is otherwise free of MRSA, and when the cost of nosocomial spread may be high. The latter is a contentious issue, but the debate serves to crystallize the logic, science, and behaviour associated with infection control (Note: many institutions use Contact Isolation for MRSA, and yet others may not use any precautions when the patient is only a carrier. There is considerable variability in the latter. It boils down to the same old question - how much effort do you want to endure to contain an infectious disease?). Some facilities would never have sufficient resources to invoke such a stringent approach. Although some exotic infections may not truly be as infectious as portrayed in lay press (e.g., Ebola virus), Strict Isolation may be applied in a circumstance where small margins of error are unacceptable.

Protective Isolation

Also known as Reverse Isolation, this technique is used to protect the patient rather than the visitor from infection. In this circumstance, clean filtered air is provided to the isolation room through **positive pressure ventilation** and is subsequently exhausted outside of the room. In this case, the patient is extremely compromised, usually from a severe lack of immunity, and it is desirable to reduce the microbial burden which the patient may be exposed to from the environment or from other individuals. For example, patients who are in the midst of bone marrow transplantation may be extremely immunocompromised and run the risk of rare but potentially lethal fungal infections such as aspergillosis. Patients with large surface areas of third-degree burns may benefit from Protective Isolation, although the actual impact of infection control measures may be debated.

Apart from positive pressure ventilation, if available, entrants to the patient's room are required to mask, glove, and gown. Essentially, the isolation has many fundamental similarities to conditions in an operating room theatre.

Whereas the above represent major isolation techniques, it is conceivable that variations on these themes will be advocated for specific infections or depending on the resources available. The methods employed must sufficiently reduce or abolish risk to an acceptable level.

The Worthy Isolation Room

Defining the essential components of a worthy isolation room is more easy than coping with the reality of existing resources. All too often, health care facilities have been designed with less concern about infection control needs, and the health care team may be left with the necessity to make the best with the least. Nevertheless, many of the fundamental needs are not difficult to include in new building or for that matter renovations.

Isolation rooms should be freely accessible but capable of closure with easily handled doors. The provision of space will depend on whether the room is intended for single patient or multi-patient areas. As previously indicated, it may be quite acceptable to quarantine more than one patient with a common illness in a sufficiently-sized room. If multi-patient use is intended, there should be sufficient space to allow for patient segregation. Any such room should be constructed to be inclusive of families and/or visitors.

Given the need to decontaminate working surfaces, the room should maintain minimum essential components and storage space for materials that should remain clean and uncontaminated. Floors, counters, beds, and other contents should be constructed so that cleaning methods are facilitated.

Ventilation needs should be considered and the majority of such needs dictate the use of negative pressure ventilation. Appropriate air exhaust is also of concern. Washroom facilities should be available in each room, and separate facilities are preferable for each patient. Sinks for handwashing are best placed inside the room, although it may also be desirable to have handwash facilities outside of rooms in particular circumstances. Soap dispensers and isolation garb must be strategically placed to maximize compliance and prevention. Safe disposal of sharps, biological waste, and other materials are essential.

Since patients may be confined to a closed room, the wall adjacent to the corridor would benefit from a see-through glass which facilitates observation by health care personnel. Signs which succinctly denote requisite isolation techniques should be posted in areas that maximize visibility for medical staff and visitors. The availability of staff to instruct visitors and patients is equally important.

Specimen Handling, Equipment, and Linens

Patient specimens, whether for the purpose of microbial diagnostics or otherwise, should all be considered as having the potential for causing human infection. Respect should be had for all such specimens as a basic standard; additional concerns may be raised when the nature of some specimens indicates added hazard. For example, liquid specimens pose the added risk of leakage from even the more highly proofed containers. Each specimen must be appropriately labelled, and the method of containment for transport should suit the specific need. In this regard, the use of pneumatic tubes for specimen transport must not be taken lightly. Well-designed protocols for transport and handling of specimens in such systems are imperative, and ultimately, these systems may be applied to a few choice specimens. Specimens should ultimately be discarded with appropriate biohazardous waste.

Equipment and medical paraphernalia are sure intermediates for the transient carriage of infectious agents. Commonly, these objects have been contaminated by hand. The microbes may remain on such inanimate objects for a variable period of time which will be influenced by the initial inoculum of germ, the nature of the surface, environmental conditions, and the presence of associated debris (e.g., mucous) from the source. The design of such materials should include a consideration for easy decontamination. The choice of ancillary objects for patients' rooms (e.g., toys for children), should also be considerate of infection control needs. Medical devices that are intended for single use should be appropriately discarded, and a general policy/protocol for decontamination of multi-use objects should be available.

Soiled linens should be maintained and then transported in impervious bags. In an era of increasing antimicrobial resistance, concerns have been raised regarding the remainder of germs on linens after routine detergent washing. It does not appear that the return of cleaned linens poses a threat in this regard when standard washing procedures are applied. Nevertheless, steamed pressing (heat) of linens does add another measure of decontamination to the latter.

Cost-Containment in an Era of Restraint

Balancing the cost and benefit of infection control procedures is often a difficult task, but it must be recognized as well that cost-benefit analyses in most medical contexts are commonly subjects for great debate. Overall, the area of cost-benefit for infection control practice is understudied, but the reasons for this may highly relate to the inability to accurately measure impact. It is much easier to calculate cost-benefit on a theoretical basis after using figures for material and labor costs and balancing them with the projected costs of hospital days and incidence of the infection. It is more difficult to design rigid and comprehensive studies which determine real costs. Indeed, the numbers of observations or patients that are required to test a hypothesis could number into the thousands. In a global sense, health outcomes can be very difficult to measure. It may be very obvious in some circumstances that a simple measure prevents infection, and thus the measure is implemented (e.g., proper decontamination of re-usable medical instruments), but there are procedures for which cost-benefit would be need to be proven (e.g., frequency of floor washing in a hospital). In so determining cost-benefit, will there be an exact dividing line between overachieving and underachieving? Given the complexity of medical care, it becomes apparent that the "level playing field" for any assessment has ongoing cycles of bumps and grinds.

It is with the aforementioned uncertainty that infection control procedures most often favour a more cautious, albeit not definitively proven, approach. It may well be that a seemingly expensive approach prevents very few adverse incidents, but it may also very well be that these uncommon incidents are considerably impactful regarding resources, morbidity, or mortality.

Less recognized is the fact that the benefit of infection control practices may be indirect rather than direct. The indirect benefits may in large part translate into the development of a mind-set or "culture" which is not complacent about the role of infection control in day-to-day activities. For example, a role for gowning on entry to a neonatal intensive care unit may be rightfully questioned if the measures are solely to be cost of gowns versus direct infections prevented. The gowning, however, may actively be a part of an overall process which seeks to prevent infection by any means. The gowning may be the adjunctive measure which prompts health care workers and visitors to more likely behave in ways that promote prevention (e.g., a stimulus to handwashing, cohorting, ensuring aseptic technique where appropriate, etc). When gowning or other seemingly low benefit manoeuvres are removed, the "culture" of infection control has a tendency to deteriorate to such an extent that even critical infection control practices are in jeopardy. Obviously, those indirect benefits may be hard to justify or prove to the more unbelieving of individuals. Just as life is a seesaw, adherence to infection control techniques wavers; more adherence in times of trouble and less adherence when everything seems to be going well.

Barriers to the Implementation of Infection Control Techniques

We may have good intentions at the best of times, but human condition is open to failure. More deliberately we can admit that the compromise in implementing infection control techniques may be a function of lack of knowledge and training or mere ignorance. We can rationalize failure on the basis of perceived costs, user-unfriendliness, and perhaps the complacency given the actual low frequency of infections. Some procedures may appear complex to some, and others may simply blame a lack of recall in a context where many other aspects of good medical care seem more deserving of attention. In addition, however, there may be a problem with what one might label as 'rebellion primacy'. The imposition of standards which may seem strict, or to some unjustified given their education and context, may lead to a conscious or more likely subconscious reaction towards resistance. In large health care institutions, infection control services may be viewed as more of an authority rather than a facilitator or perhaps as a policing mechanism rather than a support. At times, it may be important to remind participants that the control of infections is of benefit to patients and all others.

Examples of barriers to infection control techniques are many, but in general these relate to impediments in the use of the basic ingredients that were earlier discussed in this chapter. Table 2 highlights give some indication of the problems in this area.

Ethics and Infection Control

As one might anticipate, infection control and its mandate touch practically all aspects of medicine. Inevitably then, there will be times when ethical issues are encountered. Since infection control must effectively deal with risk and manage it, undesirable confrontations are likely to occur more or less given the diversity of personalities and circumstances in the health care climate. These of course can be minimized, but the finding of error and its subsequent correction may fuel interpersonal discord.

We all have responsibilities of our own in the health care setting, but these fundamentally revolve about caring and securing a safe environment for patients and the public. Whereas, however, we may have an obvious view of how the conduct of good infection control should proceed, there may be circumstances where either personal or institutional responses make obstruction. An institution, for example, may be fearful of medicolegal retaliation if a problem is identified. An individual (e.g., surgeon) who is associated with a high frequency of procedure-affiliated infections, may fear medicolegal consequences, castigation amongst peers, restriction in practice, and indeed be isolated. There may also be conflicts of interest among the health care worker and the institution given that the individual works for the institution and not directly for a given patient. Thus, infection control services must have some reasonable autonomy. Those who implement good infection control should have a reasonable degree of safety in identifying risk and managing it. We must then uphold professional standards and professional ethics. Infection control implementation should be accomplished with integrity, fairness, and safety, and without bias. Coercive and suppressive responses to infection control deliberations must be met with courage and effective communication. Appropriate infection control cannot be dictated by medical politicians, fearful and unknowledgeable administrators, or threatening institutional lawyers.

Table 2. Limitations to the effective use of infection control techniques.

Handwashing
- time requirements and busy schedules
- need to re-wash (e.g., between patients)
- a lack of perceived standardization
- nature of the handwashing agent
- nature of the handwashing facility
- allergy to the handwashing agent
- availability of the handwashing facility
- re-use dermatitis

Gloving
- availability and placement
- perceived tactile limitations
- allergy to gloves
- assumption that handwashing is sufficient

Masking
- physical impediment
- heat
- fogging of eyeglass lenses
- doubt of efficacy or need
- lack of recognition that mucous membranes are a portal of entry

Gowning
- cost
- availability and placement
- physical impediment
- heat
- doubt of efficacy or need

Decontamination
- standardization of techniques
- direct cost and physical resources
- need for physical labour
- variation in surfaces (e.g., complexity, material)
- nature of the agent (e.g., toxicity, smell)
- time requisites
- allergy to decontaminating agents

Ventilation
- cost
- need for prospective planning
- problems with old buildings and existing structures
- doubt of efficacy or need

How can these working dilemmae be crystallized? One approach may be to simply practice infection control as you would like others to practice it for yourself, your family, and your friends!

Consider the Masses, Remember the Individual

With the pristine view that appropriate infection control may be beneficial for patients and others, it is easy to lose sight of possible adverse outcomes that may arise when imposing isolation precautions. For some patients, stringent precautions may lead to anxiety and perhaps depression or a variety of psychosocial stressors, especially when their enforcement is prolonged. Patients may find that there is a stigma about having been labeled with a quarantinable disease and more likely when the illness or germ carriage are chronic. Staff may be hesitant in approaching isolation rooms if not only because there is perceived to be an increased inherent workload or bother. Some patients may simply not receive the usual attention, or for that matter standard of care, because of the context. These issues do not create insurmountable barriers, however, and as human genius can create effective infection control precautions, so too can we develop patient-oriented strategies to overcome any psychosocial concerns.

Food For Thought

1. Attempt to recall the infections that you as a health care professional have encountered over the recent past. Were methods for prevention and/or quarantine implemented, and if not, would you propose any specific interventions?
2. Have there been any controversies in implementing any infection control practices in your area of work? If so, outline the nature of the controversy and specify arguments for both sides of the issue.
3. Create an architect's floor plan for a 'perfect' isolation room.
4. What benefits and disadvantages are there for wearing masks?
5. What are the manifestations of latex glove allergy?
6. What is negative pressure ventilation, and how is it achieved and standardized?
7. Explain the terminology 'Transmission-Based Precautions' and related categories of precautions. Compare them to efforts being implemented in your institution.
8. Examine your own healthcare setting. How would you best manage recommendations for the prevention of spread of: ... MRSA? ... influenza?... of a patient with *E. coli*-containing draining abscess in which the bacterium is resistant to all available antibiotics except two?

Supplemental Reading
(continuing to use the scientific medical literature)

Beggs CB, Kerr KG, Noakes CJ, Hathway EA, Sleigh PA. The ventilation of multiple-bed hospital wards: review and analysis. *American Journal of Infection Control*. Vol. 36: pages 250-259 (2008).
- why is there variation among medical institutions?

Belkin NL. The evolution of the surgical mask: filtering efficiency versus effectiveness. *Infection Control and Hospital Epidemiology*. Vol. 18: pages 49-57 (1997).
- a controversy then and now

Bolon M. Hand Hygiene. *Infectious Disease Clinics of North America*. Vol. 25: pages 21-43 (2011).
- to wash or not to wash, that is the question!

Carroll R and the American Society for Healthcare Risk Management. *Risk Management Handbook for Health Care Organizations*. 6th Edn. San Francisco, CA:Jossey-Bass A. Wiley Imprint, 2010.
- infection control is a form of risk management

Cleenewerck MB. Update on medical and surgical gloves. *European Journal of Dermatology* Vol. 20: pages 434-442 (2010).
- it will make you look at your gloves differently the next time

Eisen DB. Surgeon's garb and infection control: what's the evidence? *Journal of the American Academy of Dermatology*. Vol. 64: pages e1-e20 (2011).
- what's the evidence?

Jefferson T, Del Mar CB, Dooley L, et al. Physical interventions to interrupt or reduce the spread of respiratory viruses. *Cochrane Database of Systematic Reviews* CD006207 (2011).
- systematic review of isolation practices

Larsen E, Kretzer EK. Compliance with handwashing and barrier precautions. *Journal of Hospital Infection*. Vol. 30 (Supplement): pages 88-106 (1995).
- don't be surprised that we are less optimal than you might initially have thought

Morgan DJ, Diekema DJ, Septowitz K, Perencevich EN. Adverse outcomes with Contact Precautions: a review of the literature. *American Journal Infection Control* Vol. 37: pages 85-93 (2009).
- this is a view of isolation precautions that we often do not think of

124

Phillips S. The comparison of double gloving to single gloving in the theatre environment. *Journal of Perioperative Practice* Vol. 21: pages 10-15 (2011).
- 'best practice' is the buzz term; be analytical when you read this

Santos RP, Mayo TW, Siegel JD. Healthcare epidemiology: active surveillance cultures and contact precautions for control of multidrug-resistant organisms: ethical considerations. *Clinical Infectious Disease* Vol. 47: pages 110-116 (2008).
- what percentage of infection control is behaviour and what percentage is science?

Siegel JD, Rhinehart E, Jackson M, Chiarello L, and the Healthcare Infection Control Practices Advisory Committee. 2007 Guideline for Isolation Precautions: Preventing Transmission of Infectious Agents in Healthcare Settings.
http://www.cdc.gov/ncidod/dhqp/pdf/isolation2007.pdf
- a good resource for the details of Standard Precautions and Transmission-Based Precautions

Weber DJ, Rutala WA, Schaffner W. Lessons learned: protection of healthcare workers from infectious disease risks. *Critical Care Medicine* Vol. 38:Supplement 8 - pages 306-314 (2010).
- a good contemporary view

"... every natural science involves three things: the sequence of phenomena on which the science is based; the abstract concepts which call these phenomena to mind; and the words in which the concepts are expressed. To call forth a concept, a word is needed; to portray a phenomenon, a concept is needed. All three mirror one and the same reality."

Antoine Laurent Lavoisier
Traité Elémentaire de Chemie, 1789

VIII. Disinfection, Antisepsis, and Sterilization

Disinfection, antisepsis, and sterilization all relate to the desirable effects of neutralizing, reducing, or eliminating germs altogether. This area is potentially complex given the variations that exist in method, agent, or microbe. By '**decontamination**', we refer to a process whereby disease-causing microbes are removed.

The history of interest in this area follows the history of other topics that have been critical to infection control, and indeed aspects of antisepsis, disinfection, and decontamination essentially provided the groundwork for many of the modern infection control practices. In ancient Egyptian times, for example, it was recognized that honey had an effect to cure skin infections presumably by its antibacterial properties. Grecians were at the same time using wine or vinegar to potentiate the dressing of wounds. A role for metallic ions to inhibit microbes was suggested inadvertently when it was noted in these same ancient times that fluids which were stored in silver or copper vessels were much less likely to become spoiled in comparison to the same fluids held in pottery. Thereafter, discoveries in microbiology by many, including Pasteur and Lister (see Chapter I), provided for the detailed scientific foundation which we now accept.

Terminology

Much confusion in this area relates to terminology which has different connotations to some especially in lay circles. From an infection control perspective, these definitions are quite clearly understood to describe specific processes. **Sterilization** describes the process whereby all forms of microbes are destroyed so that the appearance of whole microbes cannot occur. The process may be physical (e.g., heat, pressurized steam) or chemical, and implies an all-or-none phenomenon. Usual sterilization processes do destroy bacterial spores (which may be relatively resistant to other methods), but they may not inactivate prions (see Chapter II) although the latter are not living forms per se. **Disinfectants** are processes, but more commonly chemical agents, which remove and reduce microbes from inanimate objects (e.g., floors, medical instruments). Disinfectants may be modestly efficient in doing so or extremely efficient and of near sterilizing capability. In this regard, it may be useful to categorize disinfectants on a spectrum of low-level to high-level of activity. The extent of disinfectant inactivation of germs will usually include many bacteria and not uncommonly some viruses and fungi. Bacterial spores are usually not fully inactivated. Some bacteria may be more susceptible than others (e.g., *M. tuberculosis* is relatively resistant to disinfectants). The intent is to eliminate pathogens from inanimate objects so that infection is minimized, but the ability of any given agent to do so varies (i.e., activity may be relative rather than absolute). The terms '**sanitizer**' and '**detergent**' are often used by the public to describe agents which have cleaning effects and which may be antimicrobial subsets of the disinfectant category. **Antiseptics** are chemical processes that are used to reduce the microbial burden on living tissue (e.g., on skin prior to surgery, e.g., handwashing agents). These usually have an intended effect on bacteria, although again viruses and fungi may be affected. The nature of antiseptics must be such that microbes are disturbed but not human tissue, and thus the antimicrobial efficacy of these agents may not be near that of more caustic and potent disinfectants. In applying either disinfectants or antisepsis to medical use, one may describe the microbial killing or microbial inhibitory activities as **germicidal** or **germistatic** respectively. Accordingly, the appropriate specific terminologies in this regard for antibacterial, antiviral, antifungal, and antispore effects are **bactericidal/bacteristatic**, **virucidal/virustatic**, **fungicidal/fungistatic**, and **sporicidal** respectively.

Outcome of Antimicrobial Processes

Whether of sterilization, disinfection, or antisepsis, there are many variables which affect the outcome of the process. These variables are dependent mainly on the microbe(s), the process, and/or the context. The specific type of microbe may vary or there may be mixtures of different microbes which vary in susceptibility. Among bacteria, resistance to these processes can be a function of spore formation, surface coats, or active methods of resistance. Viruses too may vary considerably in susceptibility (e.g., rhinoviruses and enteroviruses are similarly sized and structured, but rhinoviruses have lipid envelopes which make them more susceptible to some disinfectants). Fungi can produce spores, although these are usually more susceptible than bacterial spores. Microbes may be protected in '**biofilms**' which are organic and inorganic debris that collect as a consequence of bacterial growth and interaction with the immediate environment. It is not uncommon to see that common environmental organisms are more resistant to some processes; perhaps this is why they are more common in the hospital environment where the use of disinfectants has selected for some of them. The nature of the process (e.g., active site of chemical action for a disinfectant) may be critical, since some forms of intrinsic resistance may pre-exist. Thereafter, processes can be affected by the quantitation of the microbe, duration of process application or contact, presence of environmental factors (e.g., blood, water, mucous) which mitigate contact between process and germ, dilution of chemical agent, nature of the surface which bears the microbial burden, pH, humidity, among other things. Ultimately, the use of a process must be considered in the context and for the intended outcome. Given the potential of these variables to stress even the most seemingly advanced processes, it is imperative that a good physical cleaning of the material be had prior to the sterilization or disinfection process. Furthermore, although processes can be designed which kill or inhibit the microbe, it must be recognized that the actual mechanical wiping or cleaning has a very important role as well in removing microbes and associated debris.

What Needs What?

The use of any particular decontaminating process is balanced with the given need and risk. Appropriately then, there are a variety of processes or agents which may be suitable in different contexts (Table 1). Critical materials may require sterilization; such materials may include surgical instruments and materials which are in contact or placed in usually sterile body sites. Quite often these materials are purchased in a pre-packaged, sterile format. Sterilized disposable materials circumvent any further need for reuse sterilization. Less important interactions, labelled as semi-critical by some, may require decontaminating processes which provide **intermediate**- or **high- level disinfection**. For the latter, the materials may interact with mucous membranes, and sterilization per se is not absolutely required (e.g., endoscopy equipment, e.g., bath tubs for burn patients). Non-critical items such floors, walls, and furniture may be processed with **low-level disinfectants** since most microbes in this environment touch skin surfaces only. In a hospital setting, due consideration must be given to categorizing these needs for each context. The actual implementation of any one process may be delegated to central service and supply control centres, environmental services staff, health care workers generally, and others. Small offices and like operations often employ less trained individuals to follow through on such processes, and therefore, an enhancement

Table 1. Recommended decontamination levels for various examples in the health care setting.

Low level disinfection
> Work surfaces
> Stethoscopes
> Blood pressure apparati
> Bedpans for same patient
> Weight scales
> Floors and walls

Intermediate level disinfection
> Thermometers
> External ear equipment
> Wash tubs
> Sinks
> Hydrotherapy pools
> Bedpans between patients

High level disinfection
> Gastroscopes
> Bronchoscopes and laryngoscopes
> Sigmoidoscopes and colonoscopes
> Nasal specula
> Vaginal specula
> Tonometers

Sterilization
> Surgical instruments (including many dental)
> Implantable devices
> Ocular spatulae
> Reusable needles or similar materials (e.g., acupuncture)

of their knowledge level in this area can be vital. It is important therefore that people in general become aware of the needs when participating in health care settings.

Sterilization

A number of physical and chemical methods can be used for **sterilization**. Of those more commonly recognized by health care professionals, **autoclaving** achieves activity by increased heat as well as increased pressure (e.g., pressurized steam)(Figure 1). Although standard settings for autoclave function are commonly used (e.g., 121°C for 30 minutes in a gravity displacement sterilizer, e.g., 132°C for 4 minutes in a prevacuum sterilizer), a sterilization effect can be achieved by many variations. The exposure to autoclaving occurs in a chamber which withstands the pressurization (akin to a pressure cooker in your kitchen). There are many variations on the theme of autoclaves, and small units can be operated in offices. Dry heat (especially prolonged and over 100°C, e.g., 170°C for 60 minutes) can also be highly effective as can be boiling for a prolonged period – these are more accessible and practical methods that can be provided in ambulatory settings. Ethylene oxide gas has historically been used for similar purposes and mainly in hospitals. This gas is favourable for the sterilization of materials that are otherwise susceptible to heat. Despite the unequivocal efficacy of ethylene oxide, concerns continue to be raised about its safety and environmental impact. Instruments that are sterilized with ethylene oxide must also be aerated for many hours. Thus, alternative methods have been designed to replace ethylene oxide, and one example of the latter is based on 'ion plasma technology'. Here, hydrogen peroxide is exposed to strong electric or magnetic fields in a closed sterilization chamber at low temperatures (40-55°C). Under

Figure 1. The autoclave: a schematic of a gravity displacement type. Steam enters from the left side of the chamber, then to displace the air in a downward direction. Appropriate pressure is achieved after entry of objects through the door and sealing of the door entry.

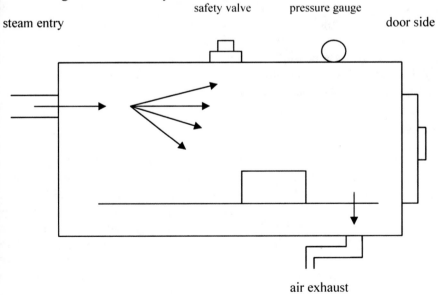

safety valve   pressure gauge

steam entry   door side

air exhaust

these conditions, an 'ion plasma' is formed in the chamber atmosphere which includes reactive free radicals that denature structures such as proteins. Not only does the latter approach circumvent ethylene oxide problems, but processing times are much shorter given the lesser requirement for aeration of sterilized instruments. Both ethylene oxide and ion plasma methods can be challenged, however, if materials, especially those reused such as surgical instruments, are not properly washed prior to sterilization. Furthermore, items with small lumens, (e.g., narrow bore endoscope channels) may also challenge the efficacy of such systems. Lastly, it is also possible to sterilize some materials by exposure to caustic or otherwise strong chemicals (e.g., glutaraldehyde), but this approach is much less often taken, and rather, such agents are used more so for high-level disinfection than sterilization. Monitoring programs for sterilization are important to ensure quality control. Specific monitors are required for different types of treatment. Manufacturer's recommendations should be heeded in order to protect instruments and other sensitive products.

Pasteurization is a form of heat processing that is reasonably active against vegetative bacteria, but it is not sporicidal. A variety of temperatures and conditions can be used as modifications of pasteurization, but it must be acknowledged that they are not substitutes for effective and proven sterilization procedures. Pasteurization has been used for some materials that are relatively heat-sensitive and that do not withstand exposure to other agents. An example of this process includes exposure to water at 75°C for 30 minutes. Pasteurization should be thought of as a form of disinfection rather than sterilization.

There are many factors which affect the workings of sterilization techniques. Residual proteins and salts and biomass can reduce penetration. Large numbers of germs and their associated biofilm accumulation affect efficacy. Some germs may be more resistant than others. Equally important is the design of the material to be decontaminated (e.g., narrow lumen instruments or lengthy lumen instruments tend to be more resistant).

Disinfection

Disinfection is a critical process in the everyday life of health care settings. Even in the home, sanitizers represent one variation on this theme. There are many different agents that can be effective disinfectants, but it must be accepted that they provide disinfection with varying degrees of efficacy. Hence, each situation of disinfectant use must consider the options of disinfectants and then deem appropriate one or few options. From the health care workers' perspective, it is often useful to narrow the selection to a few disinfectants that span the needs of low-, intermediate-, and high-level disinfection; otherwise, it may be very confusing to some when many choices are made available. Among this broad group of agents, some of the more common include various aldehydes, alcohols, iodophors, phenolics, chlorine-based compounds, acids and alkalis, biguanides, triclosan, quaternary ammonium compounds, detergents, and hydrogen peroxide. This is but a partial list of a very complex area.

In addition to the use of single agents, there are various combinations of these which may be equally or more effective. In part, some combinations are created with the intent of reducing higher concentrations of single agents. Nevertheless, it is imperative at times to observe minimum effective concentrations for some chemicals. It cannot be over-stated that instruments and materials must be properly cleaned prior to disinfection since, like sterilization, any process can be overcome if the conditions are sufficiently conducive. In the current era, most manufacturers of re-usable medical supplies have predetermined the examples of effective and tolerable disinfectants. Materials such as glass lenses and their respective adhesives, plastic or similar malleable materials, and metal alloys often present the greatest challenge. In addition, microsurgery and advanced endoscopic methods have driven the need for instruments with very narrow lumena which may prove difficult to clean. As chemical agents, usually in solution, are re-used, they become susceptible to dilution and evaporation which can alter the effective working concentrations. Regard to expiry dates and minimum effective dilutions and concentrations is critical. Working or higher dilutions can be toxic to human tissue, and toxicity profiles should be available and understood. There may be some contexts where toxicity is a concern and yet others where controlled conditions mitigate such concerns (e.g., glutaraldehyde use in open containers in a non-ventilated room versus glutaraldehyde use in an automated washer).

The following discussion provides highlights for some common agents but is not an endorsement for any particular agent or process. Again, the choice of disinfectant must meet the needs of the task.

Aldehydes

Formaldehyde is an example of such a compound, but its use for disinfection is now limited in large part due to concerns that were raised about hazards in the workplace. It is mainly used as a fixative for surgical tissue prior to microscopic analysis. **Glutaraldehyde** is nevertheless commonly used. Its use is advocated in a 2% solution, and it is particularly suited to use as an aqueous high-level disinfectant. For example, it is commonly used for disinfecting endoscopy equipment. This agent non-specifically alters the structure of numerous cellular constituents including proteins and genetic material. It has good tuberculocidal action and is reasonably sporicidal for some spores such as those of *Clostridium difficile*. Exposures of 20-30 minutes at room temperature generally suffice. Care should be taken to minimize dilution of the original 2% solution if re-use is contemplated. Vapors of glutaraldehyde are a problem to health care workers, and hence the product should be used in areas where ventilation is sufficient. Contact dermatitis is a major problem for some repetitive handlers. Overall, this agent has retained a place in disinfection mainly due to its proven efficacy where other time-honoured processes had failed. Newer aldehyde variations are becoming available, but their use must follow the limitations indicated by the manufacturer. Furthermore, the use of any aldehyde product should take concern for possible effects on instruments.

Alcohols

Methanol, **ethanol**, **isopropanol**, and butanol are good antibacterials, but they are not active against spores. Their use is therefore usually restricted to low- and intermediate- level disinfection. Exposure times should be ~20-30 minutes, and effective concentrations in water range from 60 to 90%. Ethanol and isopropanol are by far the most commonly used as disinfectants and antiseptics. Exposed instruments should be dried and have allowances for evaporation prior to use. Given the volatility of alcohols, it is possible that re-use will be associated with excess dilution of the alcohol, and it must be recognized that these agents are flammable. Alcohols do not penetrate debris, and care must be taken to consider adverse impact on medical equipment especially that which contains glues and plastics. 70% isopropanol is commonly used for pre-packaged skin wipes.

Iodophors

These agents serve as low- or intermediate- level disinfectants although most use is for the purposes of antisepsis rather than disinfection. The effect of the compounds is largely through the availability of free iodine. Historically, tincture of iodine was recognized as a good antibacterial, but it was irritating and left a noticeable stain. Improvements in this area occurred when '**iodophors**' were created – carrier agents were designed which formed complexes with iodine and thereafter allow for slow release. A popular example of an iodophor is povidone-iodine (often used in solutions of 5-7.5%). Iodine acts non-specifically and interferes with a variety of cellular processes; these effects have not been especially well-characterized. Despite activity against many microbes, it is of interest that some bacteria will survive and even grow in working dilutions of iodophors. These agents should not be used in a context where newborn skin may be subject to prolonged exposure since metabolic effects are possible.

Phenolics

Phenol is a caustic chemical which was recognized as a potent disinfectant for many decades, but currently-used **phenolics** are derivatives of the same (e.g., *o*-phenylphenol, e.g., *o*-benzyl-*p*-chlorophenol). There are many different such derivatives, but most have similar antimicrobial properties. They are not sporicidal, and there has been some debate regarding their antibacterial (especially tuberculocidal) activity. They are generally used for low- or intermediate- level disinfection, and more commonly, they are applied to work surfaces such as floors or counters. Phenolics are also not uncommonly packaged in phenolic combinations or with other disinfectants. Hexachlorophene is a biphenol derivative which in the past enjoyed much use as a topical disinfectant and especially antiseptic. It is less commonly used today, and some concerns were previously raised about systemic absorption among newborns who received skin applications. Phenolics as a group are commonly components of household sanitizers. Phenolics may be irritating to the skin especially in undiluted concentrations.

Chlorine-based compounds

These agents yield free chlorine and, in the presence of water, hypochlorous acid. Solutions which achieve 1000 parts per million (ppm) of chlorine are quite active and achieve bactericidal, virucidal, fungicidal, and sporicidal potential given that the exposure time is sufficient. The most commonly used examples of these agents are **hypochlorites**, and household bleach is a solution with 5-6% sodium hypochlorite. The latter is quite conveniently available, and a 1:10 working dilution provides much more than 1000 ppm of available chlorine. The availability of free chlorine will deteriorate after dilutions of household bleach are made, and thus daily fresh dilutions are advocated. Other chlorine-based compounds may slowly release active chlorine, and these often act as household sanitizers. Chlorine compounds are widely used for disinfection and would be used even more so were it not for their corrosive action in some settings (e.g., deterioration of metals). Dilutions of household bleach are not uncommonly used to clean blood spills. Dakin's solution includes a chlorinated soda and has been used as an antiseptic for surgical wounds. Chlorine is also widely used to treat water in an effort to reduce bacterial load and eliminate pathogens. A dangerous and rapid release of chlorine gas can occur when hypochlorites are admixed with acids.

Acids and alkalis

Extremes of pH in either direction in themselves are antimicrobial, but acids and alkalis also have other direct effects on cellular constituents. Lye (sodium hydroxide) and ammonia solutions have been commonly used as household sanitizers. They are cheap and effective, but not commonly utilized in health care settings. Acetic acid is a reasonable antibacterial especially when used in concentrations that are equivalent to household vinegar (~6%). Peracetic acid in concentrations over 0.2% is a good antimicrobial, and sporicidal action can also occur to some extent. Peracetic acid breaks down as water, acetic acid, hydrogen peroxide, and oxygen. Both acids and alkalis may potentially damage a range of metals and alloys; their use in the medical setting should be carefully tailored.

Biguanides

The best known and commonly used example of this group is **chlorhexidine** which is available in several forms. Chlorhexidine is mainly used as an antiseptic, and it is active mainly against bacteria (but not bacterial spores) at 2-4% concentrations. A 0.5% solution has also been formulated in 70% alcohol.

Triclosan

Triclosan is a unique chemical which has been used as an antimicrobial since the 1960s and has been marketed in the past as Irgasan. It is believed to be safe, and it is provided in a water-based solution; the active ingredient retains activity on skin after application and washing. The chemical structure is derived from phenol but its uses are much different than other phenolics. It is mainly antibacterial and broadly affects Gram positive and Gram negative bacteria. Its action against bacteria putatively involves a variety of mechanisms. It is increasingly being used in a variety of consumer and professional products and thus mentioned in this context. It is more likely to be used on skin rather than work surfaces.

Quaternary Ammonium Compounds

Quaternary ammonium compounds are affectionately known as 'quats'. They provide low-level disinfection, and they function mainly as limited antibacterials. They are not sporicidal. Many variations of quaternary ammonium compounds have been produced, and several facets of these modifications alter the antibacterial action against specific species. They are mainly used as sanitizers for floors, walls, and counter surfaces. Interestingly, bacterial contamination of these solutions with environmental bacteria can occur, and they may not act as substrates for bacterial growth especially when the dilutions are low. Benzalkonium chloride is among the more time-honoured of these.

Detergents

Detergents are essentially surface-active agents which initially serve to solubilize lipids and other debris. As such, they are well suited for simple washing, and they facilitate the mechanical removal of unwanted soilage. Detergents have a portion of their structure which associates with water (hydrophilic) and an alternate protion which associates closer with fatty substances (hydrophobic and lipophilic). In an aqueous solution, the interaction of detergents with various materials yields 'micelles'; essentially these are dispersions of the soilage (Chapter VII, Figure 1). Detergents may also be relatively antibacterial if such activity can affect surface structures such as cell membranes. Overall, these agents are used for low-level disinfection. Like quaternary ammonium compounds, they may become contaminated with some resistant environmental bacteria. Commonly, detergents will be used as agents to facilitate handwashing.

Hydrogen peroxide

Topical use of **hydrogen peroxide** (3%) has been touted for antisepsis of wounds, but it is lesser known that similar and slightly higher concentrations can serve as disinfectants. Hydrogen peroxide produces free radicals which are believed to interact with several microbial constituents much like the effects of ozonation. Use of this agent has been hindered in part due to the recognition that several bacterial species produce enzymes (e.g., catalase) that break down hydrogen peroxide, but this appears to be overcome by high concentrations ($\geq$6%). As previously discussed, hydrogen peroxide has found its way into ion plasma sterilization. A more complete understanding of its disinfectant properties, touted by some as considerably broad, is being actively studied. Hydrogen peroxide is a strong oxidizer, and it must be stabilized in aqueous solutions.

Antisepsis

Antiseptic agents must be tolerable to the user and after repeated uses. Several of the aforementioned disinfectants may serve as antiseptics albeit at altered concentrations. In addition to the chemical effect, antisepsis is optimized by the mechanical act of cleaning or scrubbing. Many antiseptics leave residua on the site of application which provide for some lingering antibacterial action. Re-application of the same agent may further add to the local build-up of the antiseptic effect. Common antiseptic uses include handwashing in health care settings, surgical preparation of skin and mucous membranes, bath and shower antisepsis, vascular site access preparation (i.e., prior to venipuncture), urinary catheter insertion, umbilical cord cleaning, wound irrigation and cleaning, and burn protection.

Chlorhexidine, povidone-iodine, triclosan, and concentrated alcohols are examples of commonly-used antiseptics. Handwashing (see Chapter VII) application prior to surgery should include at least two minutes of scrubbing, and some may choose longer periods if the wash is the first of the day. When repetitive handwashes are required between patients over the course of the day, wash times of 20-30 seconds are practical.

Antiseptics reduce bacterial load and in some contexts quite significantly so, and they may prevent regrowth of bacteria over the initial few hours after application. They are uncommonly absolute in their decontaminating ability, however, and regrowth may occur to original numbers depending on the agent dilution and the mechanics and time of washing.

The use of antiseptics is broadening considerably, and examples of these agents are being found in household soaps, dentifrice, shampoos, shower gels, deodorants, and mouthwashes. Concerns have been expressed about whether such widespread use will have a role in promoting adverse bacterial resistance to these agents at some future date.

Evaluations of Decontaminating Processes

There are many scientific publications regarding the efficacy and comparative efficacy of antiseptics, disinfectants, and sterilants. Whereas such measures and comparisons may exist, there is often debate regarding how applicable these assessments are to real life situations. On a historic basis, many such assessments have used different techniques, and it is not difficult to make one agent seem more beneficial over another by simple alterations in the study design. Despite seemingly scientific comparisons, there are few guidelines world-wide which are acceptable to all authorities and which may be seen as minimum acceptable standards. Both science and experience are equally weighed in selecting antiseptics. Currently-used antiseptics serve as the standard for comparison.

Standardization of disinfectants, although desirable, is also fraught with difficulties because of the many conditions under which they may be used. Accordingly, methodology for assessing disinfectants vary considerably.

Sterilization is perhaps most easily monitored since the process is expected to lead to no viable remnant. In this situation, the sterilizing process should inactivate a minimum of one million bacterial spores (i.e., sterilization implies that the probability of a surviving spore is one in a million or less). Spore-laden capsules or strips (containing *Bacillus stearothermophilus* or *Bacillus subtilis* or other test germ depending on the process under assessment) are commonly used for this purpose, although enzymatic methods (i.e., heat inactivation of an enzyme) have also emerged which correlate with sterilization as indicated over a few hours. Sterility checks with spore tests are commercially available, prepackaged, and usually used as part of a routine assessment. In addition to the latter, heat sterilizers usually have temperature records which should also be monitored.

In general, it is also possible to use routine microbial cultures to assess sterility and quality of disinfection.

A Rare But Special Case

Assuming medical instruments and supplies are precleaned, contemporary sterilization procedures are highly effective in eradicating infectious agents, whether bacterium, virus, fungus, or parasite. Only special circumstances challenge these very effective processes. The same cannot be said, however, of prions (see Chapter II) which are recognized as agents of 'mad cow disease'. Examples are quite clearly documented where the responsible agent of Creutzfeldt-Jakob Disease has been transmitted during surgery (e.g., neurosurgery) after instruments, which were used on an infected patient, were subjected to standard sterilization procedures. The widespread concern of prion transmission from animal sources, especially in Europe, has added to the theoretical potential for increasing exposure to prion agents. Added to these concerns is the fact that subclinical illness may go unrecognized among some patients. In circumstances where prion transmission is a real concern, the use of disposable, single-use items that may be subject to incineration is advisable. Some have determined that the prion agent is susceptible to bleach or 1N sodium hydroxide over one hour at room temperature. Others have advocated steam sterilization of 132°C for 30 minutes to one hour, and yet others advocate a combination of alkali exposure and steam sterilization. Regardless, it is of value to have a system which provides some forewarning of high risk patients and procedures, and which activates the necessary pre-designed protocols for surgical procedure, tissue handling, and decontamination. It is certain that this topic will occupy the minds of individuals as the true impact of animal transmission to humans becomes apparent.

Food For Thought

1. Examine decontaminating products at home and at work, and determine what their active ingredients include.
2. What products are commonly used as surgical scrubs?
3. In what circumstances is it preferable to achieve sterilization rather than disinfection?
4. Toys are often found in waiting areas of health facilities. What toys facilitate the implementation of good hygiene measures?
5. What type of sterilizer exists in your workplace, and what are the principles of how it works?

Supplemental Reading

Block SS. *Disinfection, Sterilization, and Preservation.* 5th Edition. Philadelphia, PA:Lippincott Williams and Wilkins, 2001.
- a highly comprehensive and technical reference that was considered by many to be one of the most authoritative textbooks in the field. Provides plenty of bed-time reading!

Fraise A, Lambert PA, Maillard J-Y. *Russell, Hugo, & Ayliffe's Principles and Practice of Disinfection, Preservation, & Sterilization.* 4th Edition. Malden, MA:Blackwell Publishing, 2004.
- a solid and complete text

McDonnell GE. *Antisepsis, Disinfection, and Sterilization: Types, Action and Resistance.* Washington, DC:American Society for Microbiology, 2007.
- some interesting discussion regarding mechanisms of resistance for the enthusiast

McDonnell G, Burke P. Disinfection: is it time to reconsider Spaulding? *Journal of Hospital Infection* Vol. 78: pages 163-170 (2011).
- truly food for thought

Rutala WA, Weber DJ, and the Healthcare Infection Control Practices Advisory Committee. Guideline for Disinfection and Sterilization in Healthcare Facilities, 2008. Centres for Disease Control, Department of Human and Health Services, Atlanta, GA, USA, 2008.
- timely concensus guidelines with meticulous referencing

"…. the truth which [science] arrives is not that which we
can ideally comtemplate without error, but that which we may
set upon without fear …."
> William Kingdon Clifford
> *Aims and Instruments of Scientific Thought*, 1872

IX. Antibiotic Use, Abuse, and Resistance

A knowledge base in the area of antimicrobials is of value to some extent for all health care workers, but it is even more so critical for all who participate in infection control endeavours. Whereas infection control has previously, and continues to, focus on the prevention of all infections, the emphasis has increased over the last two decades towards problems which stem from the nosocomial transmission of antibiotic-resistant bacteria. In some hospitals, the battle against antimicrobial resistance is monumental and represents among the major efforts, if not the major effort, of infection control on a daily basis.

What is an Antibiotic?

Antibiotics are chemical agents which can be administered orally, systemically, or topically to patients in order to kill or inhibit microbes. They may be used to actively treat infections or to prevent some infections (i.e., prophylaxis). These agents may be quite selective in their efficacy or they may act broadly against large groups of bacteria. With some exceptions, these agents tend not to have overlapping activity against the bacterial, viral, fungal, and parasitic groups.

The term '**antibiotic**' was initially used to describe a naturally-occurring agent, especially that which was produced by some microbes. For example, penicillin was derived from the fungal mold *Penicillium*. After the discovery of these naturally-occurring agents, scientists made many modifications of the chemical structures which then altered various characteristics of these agents including spectrum of activity, absorption, distribution in the body, among other things. In addition, a number of antimicrobials were developed directly from laboratory synthesis, and these too were subjected thereafter to modifications for the benefit of medicine. In effect, all of these agents can be classified as '**antimicrobials**', whereas 'antibiotic' was coined in reference to naturally-occurring substances. Over time, however, these terms have been practically merged, and they are now essentially synonymous. Indeed, some formerly natural-source antibiotics can presently be produced synthetically.

The intent of antibiotic use is to achieve the desired antimicrobial effect while minimizing the potential toxicity to the patient. Some antibiotics are extremely safe (e.g., penicillin), and there is a very wide margin between effective and toxic doses. Some antibiotics have a much lower threshold for toxicity, and their use must be monitored in order to minimize harmful effects (e.g., therapeutic monitoring of aminoglycoside use to prevent kidney dysfunction or loss of hearing). Yet other agents may have a known and accepted toxicity which must be balanced against the need to achieve cure for an infection (e.g., some anti-HIV antivirals cause persistent metabolic changes). With regards to antibacterial agents, the spectrum of action may be narrow and reasonably directed to the infection rather non-specifically against the normal body microbial flora (e.g., some antituberculous agents). In other circumstances, it may be desirable to have an antibacterial effect that is widely active against many species or broad groups, and we refer to these agents as '**broad-spectrum antibiotics**'. An inevitable consequence of the latter, however, is that the normal microbial flora may be broadly suppressed as well.

Antibiotic Groups

In the current era, there are many antibiotic groups and several antibiotic variations within these groups more or less. In addition, many existing antibiotics have similar properties and spectra of activity. Hence, we have both a selection of equieffective antibiotics for the same purpose as well as a large armamentarium for selected requirements. Table 1 outlines this diversity in part for antibacterial agents.

Penicillin and similar antibiotics are the most commonly used both in hospital and the community. Many of these agents have also been referred to as beta-lactam agents on the basis of having a particular chemical structure (see Figure 1). Generalizing, the trend has been to create more potent antibiotics, especially those that can be used orally or that can be used against usually resistant bacteria (e.g., *Pseudomonas aeruginosa*). Others have purposely been designed to be antistaphylococcal by way of resistance to degrading enzymes (see later). Cephalosporins as a group are similar to penicillins in mode of action but have slightly different chemical structures. In the clinics, they are commonly subclassified into first, second, third, and fourth generation; these categories relate to timing of synthesis as well as some degree to their spectrum of action. Carbapenems and monobactams are further variations along the penicillin and cephalosporin theme.

Table 1. Major antibiotic groups for human therapeutic use. The listed antibiotics are only representative of a much larger armamentarium.

'Penicillins'
penicillin
ampicillin
amoxycillin
cloxacillin
piperacillin
mecillinam

Aminoglycosides
gentamicin
tobramycin
amikacin
streptomycin
framycetin
netilmicin

Folic acid antagonists
sulfonamides (many)
trimethoprim

Macrolides
erythromycin
azithromycin
clarithromycin

Various other anti-tuberculous
isoniazid
ethambutol
pyrazinamide

Monobactams
aztreonam

Cephalosporins
1st generation
   cephalothin
   cefazolin
   cephalexin
2nd generation
   cefoxitin
   cefuroxime
   cefaclor
3rd generation
   cefotaxime
   ceftazidime
   ceftriaxone
   cefixime
4th generation
   cefepime
   cefpirome

Glycopeptides
vancomycin
teichoplanin

Clindamycin

Bacitracin

Mupirocin

Polymyxins

Streptogramins
quinupristin-dalfopristin

Daptomycin

Carbapenems
meropenem
imipenem
ertapenem

Chloramphenicol

Tetracyclines
tetracycline
doxycycline
minocycline
tigecycline (a
glycylcycline)

Metronidazole

Nitrofurantoin

Rifampin

Quinolones
nalidixic acid
norfloxacin
ciprofloxacin
ofloxacin
levofloxacin
moxifloxacin

Fusidic acid

Oxazolidinones
linezolid

Figure 1. The basic structure of a penicillin molecule. The same structure with modifications is the basis for many antibiotics which resemble penicillin.

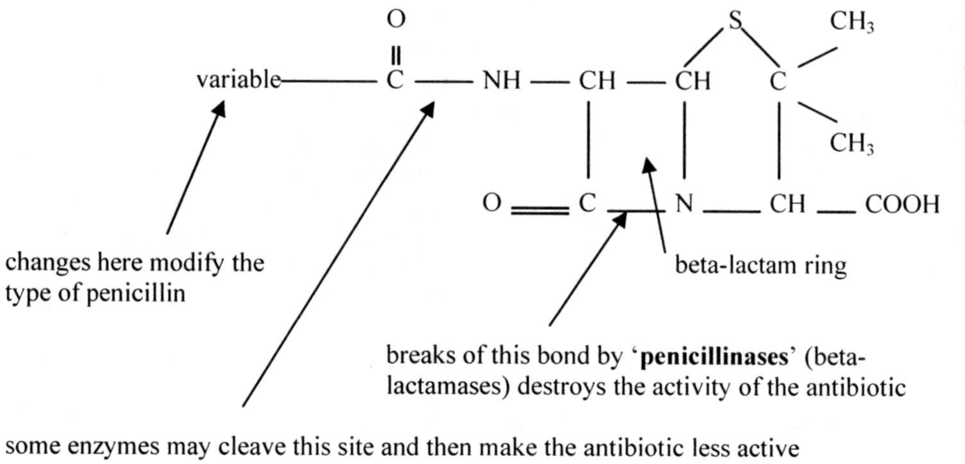

changes here modify the type of penicillin

beta-lactam ring

breaks of this bond by '**penicillinases**' (beta-lactamases) destroys the activity of the antibiotic

some enzymes may cleave this site and then make the antibiotic less active

Aminoglycosides are unique antibiotics that are used topically or intravenously, but the latter use in hospitals for serious infections is most common. Tetracyclines are not as commonly used as they once were, but they have a broad spectrum of activity. Sulphonamides and trimethoprim are differently structured, but they act on bacterial folic acid synthesis; they are mainly used to treat urinary tract infections. A combination of trimethoprim and the sulphonamide called sulphamethoxazole (referred to by some as cotrimoxazole) is quite commonly used. Macrolide antibiotics (also similar to clindamycin) are increasingly being used for out-patient therapy, and variations with less side effects, albeit more costly, are especially used in pediatric care. Quinolones initially served as urinary tract infection agents, but agents with an increased spectrum of antibacterial activity have been produced. Other antibiotics have their niche. Most antituberculous antibiotics are mainly active against mycobacteria and are not commonly used for other types of bacterial infection.

Table 2 highlights some common 'drug-bug' combinations in routine practice. There are many exceptions to these generalizations that may be dictated by the type of infection or documented antibiotic resistance. Some infections may have 'first-line', 'second-line', or 'third-line' treatments depending on ease of administration, safety, and cost.

Table 2. Antibiotics which may be commonly used to treat infections that are caused by various bacteria.

Staphylococci
cloxacillin
vancomycin
macrolides
first generation
   cephalosporins
some sulphas

Anaerobic infections
metronidazole
clindamycin
some advanced penicillins
some advanced
   cephalosporins
carbapenems

Legionella
erythromycin

Enterococci
ampicillin

Gram negative bacilli
of enteric origin
advanced penicillins
cephalosporins
aminoglycosides
quinolones
folic acid antogonists

Chlamydiae
macrolides
tetracyclines

Mycoplasmas
macrolides
tetracyclines

Streptococci
penicillins
cephalosporins
macrolides
vancomycin

Pseudomonas and similar
bacteria
advanced cephalosporins
advanced penicillins
aminoglycosides
advanced quinolones

Rickettsiae
tetracyclines
chloramphenicol

Bordetella pertussis
erythromycin

Table 3 outlines common antiviral, antifungal, and antiparasitic agents. Again, these combinations are provided for the purposes of illustrating commonalities, but there are several exceptions and many other examples under some of these categories.

Mechanisms of Action

Antibacterials

Despite the many available antibiotics and despite some variations in the detail of how agents from the same group may exert their effect, there are a few generalizations which summarize how they work (Figure 2). Penicillins, cephalosporins, carbapenems, monobactams, and glycopeptides interfere with the creation of the bacterial cell wall. For example, penicillin binds to so-called **penicillin-binding proteins** which are integral to such cell wall synthesis. An interrupted cell wall will allow for the bacterium to lyze under particular environmental circumstances.

144

Table 3. Examples of antimicrobials that are used to treat viral, fungal, and parasitic infections.

Antiviral

<u>Influenza agents</u>
amantidine
rimantidine
oseltamivir
zanamivir

<u>anti-cytomegalovirus</u>
ganciclovir
foscarnet

<u>hepatitis C</u>
interferon-alfa
ribavirin

<u>respiratory syncytial virus</u>
(controversial efficacy)
ribavirin

<u>anti-Herpes simplex and</u>
<u>anti-Herpes zoster</u>
acyclovir
famciclovir
valacyclovir

<u>papillomavirus</u>
imiquimod
interferon-α-2b

<u>HIV</u>
zidovudine
lamivudine
indinavir
nevirapine
didanosine
zalcitabine
stavudine
saquinavir
vitonavir
enfuvirtide

<u>hepatitis B</u>
lamivudine

Antifungal

<u>topical use</u>
tolnaftate
ciclopirox
clotrimazole
nystatin
ketoconazole
terbinafine

<u>oral or systemic use</u>
amphotericin B   caspofungin
5-flucytosine   ketoconazole
terbinafine
fluconazole
itraconazole
voriconazole

Antiparasitic

<u>antiamoebic</u>
metronidazole
iodoquinol

<u>antimalarial</u>
chloroquine
mefloquine
primaquine
doxycycline
atovaquone/proguanil

<u>anti-*Pneumocystis*</u>
sulfa-trimethoprim
pentamidine

<u>deworming</u>
mebendazole
pyrvinium
pyrantel pamoate
albendazole

Other antibiotics (e.g., polymyxins) interact with the cell membrane rather than cell wall and effectively poke holes in its integrity. A number of antibiotics (e.g., macrolides, clindamycin, tetracyclines, aminoglycosides) actively interfere with the synthesis of cellular proteins through a variety of

Figure 2. Sites of action of common antibacterial agents.

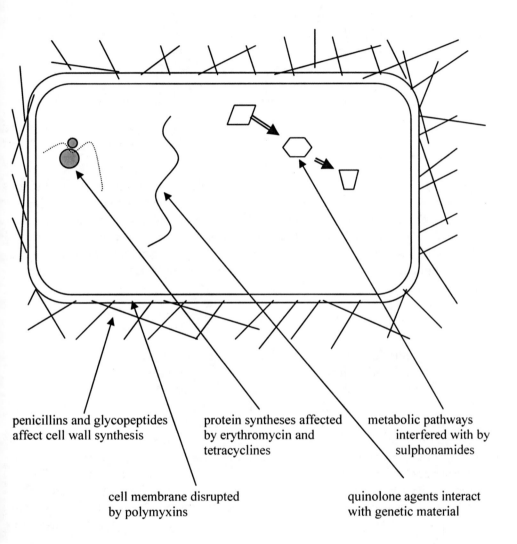

penicillins and glycopeptides
affect cell wall synthesis

protein syntheses affected
by erythromycin and
tetracyclines

metabolic pathways
interfered with by
sulphonamides

cell membrane disrupted
by polymyxins

quinolone agents interact
with genetic material

mechanisms. One of the more common examples of the latter is to interfere with the function of ribosomes which act as sites for protein templates. Several antibiotics (e.g., quinolones, sulphas, trimethoprim) interfere with the replication of genetic material by way of direct interference or in the pathway of developing building blocks.

Antivirals

Antiviral agents tend to be less broadly acting in contrast to a potent antibacterial. Some antivirals inhibit the multiplication of viruses that are inside of human cells either through activity against their genetic replication or through inhibition of viral proteins. Others may affect the virus' attachment to and uncoating within cells. Yet others may work to change the body's immune response. With the need to provide effective anti-HIV therapy, new targets for anti-viral agents are quickly emerging.

Antifungals and Antiparasitics

Both fungi and parasites are eukaryotic microbes. With such a higher evolutionary scale, their cellular machinery and physical structures are much different and indeed more complex. Both antifungals and antiparasitics are quite diverse in their mechanisms of action. There are many variations regarding antibiotic and microbe combinations. The similarity of some cellular elements to those of human cells explains why the margin between efficacy and toxicity may be small.

What Determines Antimicrobial Use?

Whether an antibiotic may be used as well as the type, route, and length of administration is influenced by many factors which most often require clinical decision-making processes. Antibiotics may be used for active treatment and prevention, although exposure to antibiotics or the consequences of use (e.g., resistance) can also occur due to veterinary needs (e.g., animal feed). The clinical presentation of an illness as well as clinical changes thereafter may indicate that an antibiotic is required. More definitive identification of a given pathogen in a particular context as well as the susceptibility testing if available will also highly influence the use of antibiotics. Of course not all infections require antibiotic therapy (e.g., a bacterial meningitis most certainly will, but a superficial skin infection, whether staphylococcal or streptococcal, may not require any antibiotics at all).

The site and seriousness of infection will bias the selection of particular agents and furthermore, the route by which they are administered. Antibiotics which are given parenterally either cannot be absorbed by oral dosing or may be needed to achieve high circulating blood levels. In turn, high blood levels correlate with increasing probability that the antibiotic will penetrate sufficiently to the site of infection. Some antibiotics may cross anatomic barriers (e.g., blood-brain barrier, e.g., abscess cavities) better than others.

Underlying and complicating illnesses may affect antibiotic choices given the potential for some antibiotics to be impacted by issues such as renal or hepatic dysfunction. As well, other pharmacological agents may affect antibiotic function and vice versa.

Other factors which influence the use and choice of antibiotics include existing immune compromise, need for broad spectrum versus narrow spectrum agents, age and pregnancy contraindications, adverse effects profiles and other general considerations, and cost.

Combinations of antibiotics may be used to treat difficult infections (e.g., tuberculosis), increase the antimicrobial spectrum of activity, reduce the potential for some antimicrobial resistances, and provide for synergistic effects. For example, combinations of beta-lactam agents and aminoglycosides are often favoured for serious Gram negative bacterial infections.

The use of prophylactic, or preventative antibiotics, has gained favour in many circumstances (Table 4). Many of these uses are for the prevention of specific infections, while others are intended to generally prevent bacterial infections.

Overall, antibiotic use should be guided by scientific verification of use and benefit. Regimens for type of antibiotic and pattern of use are well-documented in many references. Experience also has a large role to play.

Problems of Use and Abuse

The discussion of antibiotic resistance certainly includes a recognition of the role that antibiotic use has in promoting said resistance. A limited and approved use of an antibiotic for the necessary treatment of an infection carries with it the risk of antimicrobial resistance developing either for the intended microbe or as a consequence of other bacteria (e.g., normal flora) evolving resistance even though they are not targeted in the treatment process. In this case, the peril was realized despite the best effort of the clinician to limit antibiotic use. On the other hand, antibiotic resistance could emerge as a consequence of excessive antibiotic use where the intent of use was nevertheless believed by the user to be correct. For example, in the area of animal husbandry, antibiotics may be used by the producer of feed animals to promote survival of newborns, increase weight gain, and prevent herd outbreaks. While the latter has obvious benefits for the farmer, a negative impact for society could be the spread of antibiotic-resistant germs from animal source to humans. In the extreme, antibiotics may be frankly abused in a context where they are administered purposely for a condition where benefit

Table 4. Some indications for the use of prophylactic antibiotics.

Antibiotic	Indication
rifampin	contacts of patients with invasive *N. meningitidis* infection
erythromycin	contacts of patients with whooping cough
penicillin or erythromycin	contacts of patients with diphtheria
penicillin	contacts of patients with invasive *S. pyogenes* infection
various regimens	pre- and intra- operative prophylaxis after major bowel surgery
various regimens	malaria prophylaxis when entering and exiting from endemic areas
various regimens	Caesarian section except in elective uncomplicated cases
various regimens	hysterectomy surgery
first-generation cephalosporins	joint replacement surgery
various regimens	appendectomy
various regimens	major surgery of head, mouth, and neck when the approach is through the oral mucosa
first-generation cephalosporins	some major cardiovascular surgeries

is recognized as minimal if any (e.g., antibiotic prescriptions for the uncomplicated cold). Whereas many forms of antibiotic use are not within the direct mandate of infection control to consider, others (especially in health care facilities) are more in the line of infection control to assess. Table 5 highlights some problems with antibiotic use that favour the development of resistance.

Table 5. Factors that favour the development of antimicrobial resistance.

- the activity spectrum of the antibiotic is overly broad
- antibiotic therapy is prolonged beyond the need
- antibiotic prophylaxis is prolonged beyond the period of true risk
- combination therapy is used although not required
- the overlapping spectrum of activities is not understood for multiple antibiotic use
- errors in judgement regarding the underlying illness and the appropriate antibiotic if any
- frank lack of knowledge regarding the specific antibiotic use
- use of empiric antibiotic treatments
- lack of relevant and practical information for new agents
- perception that urgent treatment is required
- perception that antibiotics are simple to use and generally lack toxicity
- dosing errors
- use for non-bacterial infections (e.g., viral origin)
- using antibiotics that are unable to satisfactorily penetrate the site of infection (e.g., abscesses, e.g., intracellular, e.g., biofilm development, e.g., infection in a blood clot)
- institutionalized care which is associated with greater proximity of patients and greater antibiotic use per capita
- patient-directed use and re-use
- incomplete diagnostic data
- lack of antibiotic regulatory structure (e.g., over-the-counter availability)
- topical versus other use
- using first choice antibiotics versus alternate or reserve antibiotics
- veterinary use
- public pressure and expectations
- industry pressure and lures
- urge to follow new trends

Mechanisms of Resistance

Resistance to antimicrobials can occur across all four broad groups of microbes. Our discussion herein focuses on bacterial antibiotic resistance, because it is by far the most common and worrisome. Viral resistance has been documented among some herpes simplex virus isolates (e.g., resistance to acyclovir usually after prolonged use), but HIV is perhaps the best example of a virus that has eluded many antiviral agents due to the frequent evolution of resistance. Antifungal resistance has been documented among yeast which have been exposed chronically during the course of antifungal prophylaxis (e.g., to prevent recurrent thrush in AIDS patients). In the area of parasitology, one of the best and most important examples is the development of drug-resistant malaria which has implications for both prevention and treatment.

Generalizing, one can understand that mechanisms of resistance follow naturally when change or barriers occur to the aforementioned mechanisms of antibiotic action. There is usually one such change or barrier which promotes resistance for a given microbe, but several mechanisms of resistance may be present at the same time. Many bacteria naturally have certain forms of antibiotic resistance (Table 6) which may have existed even prior to the advent of antibiotics. The acquisition of additional resistance profiles has largely occurred due to the exposure of these bacteria to the given antibiotic over time. If resistance did not evolve above and beyond the inherent resistances that are exemplified in Table 6, we would be able to cope given the realized potential to synthetically create antibiotics that overcome these forms of resistance. It is the subsequent acquisition of resistance by several means that has proven to be very difficult to contend with.

Table 6. Examples of common antimicrobial resistances that are inherent (intrinsic) to various bacteria.

Gram positive bacteria	-	polymyxins
Gram negative bacteria	-	glycopeptides
Anaerobic bacteria	-	aminoglycosides
Enterococcus spp.	-	anti-staphylococcal penicillins, cephalosporins
Listeria spp.	-	cephalosporins
Escherichia coli and other coliforms	-	narrow spectrum penicillins, anti-staphylococcal penicillins
Neisseria gonorrhoeae	-	trimethoprim, polymyxin
Pseudomonas aeruginosa	-	narrow spectrum penicillins, 1st & 2nd generation cephalosporins
Clostridium difficile	-	cephalosporins
Campylobacter jejuni	-	cephalosporins

All organisms, eukaryotic or procaryotic, have the potential to mutate. A **mutation** in the genetic material of a bacterium may lead to antibiotic resistance when the change alters the product of a given gene. The subsequent alteration may render an active site of the antibiotic less vulnerable. It is also possible that the mutation changes the regulation of other genes that are instrumental in producing antibiotic-degrading enzymes. Some resistance genes may be innately present, but they may be relatively silent until they are 'switched on'. This switching can occur as a function of exposure to the antibiotic or by changes in regulatory genes. In addition to mutations of the bacterium's genetic make-up, bacteria may acquire new genetic material which brings the resistance genes with it. The latter can occur by several mechanisms as shown in the Figure 3. These mechanisms include: a) transport into the cell by bacterial viruses, b) uptake of bacterial DNA directly from the environment (this DNA may have been derived from another resistant bacterium), c) transfer of highly mobile genetic elements call **plasmids** (these are usually circular bits of DNA that are present in addition to the main single chromosome), and d) transfer of highly mobile genetic elements called **transposons** ('jumping genes') which are able to move back and forth between chromosome and plasmids. When new genetic material which confers resistance is acquired by a bacterium, it must have acquired it from a particular source. The latter source is usually a pre-existing resistance in a similar organism.

The acquisition of resistance may be fortuitous and occur within a short period of time. Mutations are spontaneous events that occur frequently. In the presence of the antibiotic, selective pressure will facilitate the growth of the resistant bacterium in contrast to the one that is susceptible. It is often somewhat unpredictable, however, as to when a patient may acquire a resistant bacterium, since there are many risk factors for such acquisition.

The major mechanisms of resistance include the following. The elaboration of enzymes that destroy or change an antibiotic is common. The most common of these destroy penicillin and similar antibiotics by the opening of the beta-lactam chemical ring. Hence, they are referred to as **beta-lactamases**. Beta-lactamases come in many different forms, and their specificity can be variable for the different beta-lactam antibiotics. A good example of the latter is the beta-lactamase of *S. aureus* which confers resistance to penicillin. Antibiotics which are resistant to this beta-lactamase degradation have been developed (e.g., cloxacillin, e.g., methicillin). Beta-lactamases with a broad spectrum of activity against many beta-lactam agents have proven to be a modern scourge. Other enzyme-based modifications of antibiotics are also possible and these include modifications by the addition of structures to the molecule of antibiotic (e.g., enzymatic modification of chloramphenicol and aminoglycosides). Other mechanisms of resistance may include changes in the outer membrane of Gram negative bacteria (functioning to exclude certain antibiotics), decreased active uptake of some antibiotics into the cell (e.g., with aminoglycosides), changes in the target of the antibiotic (e.g., decreased affinity for an antibiotic when the binding proteins are altered, or alteration in the ribosomal target for some antibiotics), and alterations in the metabolic synthetic pathway that may be interfered with by a class of antibiotics (e.g., folic acid synthesis impeded by sulpha drugs and trimethoprim).

Figure 3. Mechanisms by which genetic information either changes or is acquired in order to generate antimicrobial resistance.

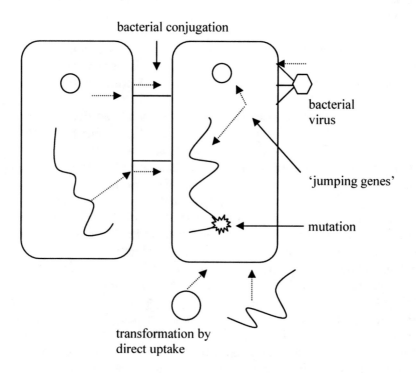

How Do We Measure Susceptibility to an Antibiotic?

Although some antibiotic use will be based on a best estimate in a given scenario, it is obviously preferable in every circumstance to tailor the antibiotic use to a specific need. The latter would impact on cost, efficacy, complications, and antibiotic resistance among other things. When the specific infecting microbe(s) is (are) known as determined by a diagnostic method (see Chapter IV), a microbe-specific antibiotic can be prescribed. If the micro-organism is routinely susceptible to an antibiotic, then specific susceptibility testing does not need to be performed. If, however, it is recognized that the antimicrobial susceptibility is variable, then a determination of the same should be performed in the laboratory if it is feasible. In general, antibiotic susceptibility testing is performed for bacteria that are easily cultivated (e.g., *S. aureus*, coliform Gram negative bacilli, enterococci, pseudomonads), but it may be exceptionally cumbersome for others (e.g., mycoplasmas, chlamydiae, rickettsiae, spirochetes, fastidious anaerobes). Furthermore, susceptibility testing should be completed and the results available on a timely basis in order for antibiotic use (and hence patient care) to be positively impacted. This information may also lead one to correct a regimen which was given empirically with best intention but which proves to be in error; exceptions and unusual patterns of illness do occur. Although methods exist, it is generally accepted that '**susceptibility testing**' (some call it 'sensitivity testing') is less well standardized and even cumbersome to perform for viruses, fungi, and parasites. The latter may change in the near future as molecular methods become more widely available. Routine susceptibility testing as we commonly know it applies mainly to a subset of rapidly-growing bacteria, and hence we discuss the methods herein.

Overall, the intent of susceptibility testing is to assess the interaction of bacterium and antibiotic in order to determine whether an antibiotic is likely to succeed in effecting cure. It must be realized that such testing provides an estimate of the probability that an outcome will occur often using an antibiotic in a given context, but it is not an absolute indicator. The actual outcome of antibiotic use will be determined by a number of factors in addition to antibiotic susceptibility testing; which of these variables most influences a particular outcome may change from patient to patient.

The specific methods that are commonly used for susceptibility testing have been subject to considerable study, and they are the result of much fine-tuning that has come about over several decades. These methods may be manual, semi-automated, or fully automated. Variations of susceptibility testing methods are generally in agreement, but some approaches may be more preferable than others for given bacteria. In each of these, the bacterial growth is assessed against a standard of antibiotic concentrations, and the ability of the bacterium to grow, or its inhibition, determine whether the bacterium is susceptible or resistant. The most commonly used methods include disk diffusion, broth microdilution (or similar compact variations), agar dilution, and Etest®.

Disk diffusion

A small paper disk is impregnated with a single antibiotic. The disk is applied to a standard agar medium which has been over-laid with the bacterium. After an incubation period that allows for the bacterium to grow fully, the degree of antibiotic susceptibility is determined by the magnitude of the diameter of inhibition of bacterium about the disk (Figure 4). Zones of inhibition have been pre-determined which correlate with sufficient susceptibility. Each antibiotic that is tested must be done so with a unique disk.

Broth microdilution

A broth culture medium is made into series of dilution wells which have ranging concentrations of the given antibiotic (Figure 5). Each of these is incubated with the bacterium to be tested. A determination is made as to whether the bacterium

Figure 4. Disk diffusion susceptibility testing.

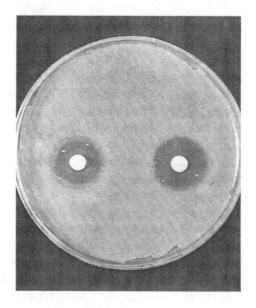

Figure 5. Broth microdilution susceptibility testing. Each circular well represents the exposure of a standard amount of bacterium to a dilution of a particular antibiotic. In this case, each horizontal row represent doubling dilutions of an antibiotic, from lesser concentration on the left to stronger concentrations on the right. The dots in each well are growths of the bacterium. Concerning the first horizontal row, there is bacterial growth in the first two wells but not in the last four. The well without growth signals the minimum amount of antibiotic that is required in the test tube to inhibit the bacterium. In the 2nd, 3rd, 5th, and 6th horizontal rows, all wells show growth dots, and thus the bacterium is resistant at all concentrations for these different antibiotics.

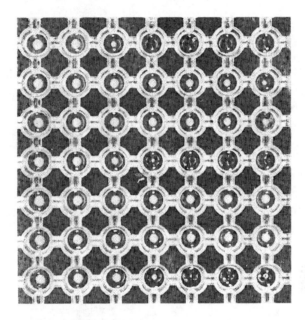

will grow in all or any. A specific dilution of antibiotic will correlate with the susceptible or resistant category. Definition of the latter will be standardized for a particular method of broth microdilution, but these determinations generally depend on the anticipated blood levels of antibiotic regardless of administration route. Variations on this theme have been automated, and numerous microdilution chambers can be fit into computer cards that are smaller than the palm of a hand. The computer will have a sensor that interprets growth or no growth in each tiny antibiotic chamber. Such automation facilitates throughput and possibly timeliness.

Figure 6. Agar dilution susceptibility testing.

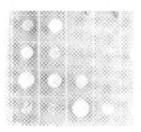

Agar dilution

A standard agar medium is made which has a specified concentration of antibiotic. The bacterium is spotted onto a portion of this medium. After an incubation period, the spot of bacterium will grow into a large colony, or there will be no growth (Figure 6). The latter correlates with resistance or susceptibility respectively. The concentration of antibiotic will be a critical one which has been pre-determined as the suitable end-point.

Etest®

This is a commercial and innovative method which is analogous to disk diffusion in many ways. Rather than using an antibiotic-laden disk, a long paper strip is impregnated with a variable and increasing concentration of antibiotic (Figure 7). Growth of the bacterium will intersect the strip in elliptical configuration and thereby indicate the relative susceptibility in a quantitative fashion.

Figure 7. Etest® diffusion susceptibility testing.

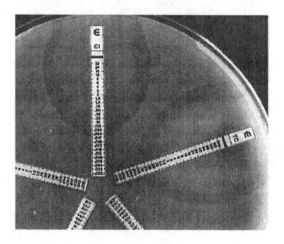

Infection control programs may use the results of these assessments to track concerning trends. In part, a susceptibility profile to many antibiotics may at times mimic a fingerprint to indicate whether isolates of the bacterium are in common.

Special Considerations

MRSA

When antibiotics first became available, *S. aureus* isolates were commonly susceptible to penicillin (see Chapter XVII). Within a short time after penicillin became available, resistance to this antibiotic increased significantly, and the mechanism of resistance was production of a beta-lactamase (penicillinase; penicillin degrading enzyme). Currently most isolates of *S. aureus* produce a beta-lactamase. Although other non-beta-lactam antibiotics emerged which could be used for *S. aureus* infections, there were successful attempts at producing beta-lactam agents which were resistant to the beta-lactamase and as well possessed good anti-staphylococcal activity. Those agents are often referred to as anti-staphylococcal penicillins and include such agents as methicillin, cloxacillin, nafcillin, and flucloxacillin. Nevertheless within a short while after these agents were utilized, resistance to them was documented, and as a group, the isolates were referred to as '**methicillin-resistant *Staphylococcus aureus***' (**MRSA**). Rather than an enzymatic destruction of the antibiotic, the new resistance mechanism involved a change in the affinity of the antibiotic for its target site of action (so-called 'penicillin-binding protein').

Whereas MRSA were uncommon in the 1960s and 1970s, they became quite prominent in the last two decades. Such resistance is now essentially a world-wide phenomenon, but some medical centres have had especially major problems with nosocomial spread. In addition to the actual resistance to anti-staphylococcal penicillins, some strains have acquired resistance to many other antibiotics. Often this acquisition has been incremental as other agents have been used for treatment, and hence the bacterium has the opportunity to meet and beat new challenges. Given the potential to possess mechanisms of resistance to a large number of antibiotics, there are very few options at times for treatment; intravenous vancomycin is commonly a preferred agent for serious infections.

As might be anticipated, the frequent use of vancomycin for this and other purposes has led to the emergence of vancomycin-intermediate resistance among *S. aureus* (so-called **VISA**). These isolates are currently rare, but still illustrate the potential consequences of antibiotic pressure. The containment of VISA, and for that matter the prevention for further progression of resistance, ultimately depends on how well we manage the MRSA issue. Since *S. aureus* is a common component of normal nasal and oral (and sometimes skin) flora, it may be difficult to eradicate.

VRE

Enterococcus spp., most notably *E. faecalis* and *E. faecium* as human pathogens, have innate antibiotic resistances to several antibiotics. For example, resistance to all cephalosporins and aminoglycosides is the norm. Some beta-lactam agents, especially ampicillin, have been principal antibiotics for enterococcal infections. Vancomycin has historically been a second-line antibiotic for this purpose. '**Vancomycin-resistant enterococci**' (**VRE**) have developed resistance to both ampicillin and vancomycin. Very few options are left for treating VRE infections, and totally new classes of antibiotics have been designed in response. VRE are currently sporadic in the community, and cross-transmission is most like to occur in hospitals especially when there is considerable antibiotic use and where there are patients who are particularly susceptible. Enterococci are commonly components of usual fecal flora, and therefore chronic carriage may in part defeat containment.

Penicillin-Resistant Streptococcus pneumoniae

S. pneumoniae is a common human pathogen which affects respiratory sites and also causes invasive infections. It is a common pediatric pathogen which especially complicates preceding viral respiratory infections. It is a major pathogen in otitis media, pneumonia, meningitis, and blood-borne infections. Historically, *S. pneumoniae* was exquisitely susceptible to penicillin, but an intermediate form of resistance became apparent especially over the last two decades. The latter has evolved into a high-level (clinical) resistance, and alongside the same, resistance to several other agents has been added. There is greatest concern for penicillin-resistant *S. pneumoniae* causing infection of the central nervous system where antibiotic penetration is marginal at the best of times.

Penicillin-resistant *S. pneumoniae* emerged in several countries but has now become a global phenomenon, although significant regional variations remain.

Multi-Resistant Coliforms

Coliform Gram negative bacilli are common components of intestinal flora and hence are often exposed to antibiotics during the treatment of other infections. They are also bacteria which easily adapt resistance profiles and are capable of maintaining one or several distinct antibiotic resistance mechanisms. This group includes *E. coli*, *Klebsiella* spp., *Enterobacter* spp., *Serratia marcescens*, *Citrobacter* spp., among others. In hospital settings, and in the era where multiple potent antibiotics may be used simultaneously, there is an emerging trend towards the development of resistance to aminoglycosides (often plasmid-borne) and to advanced broad-spectrum beta-lactam agents. Some isolates, for example, have developed resistance to penicillin, cephalosporins, monobactams, and carbapenems. The latter resistance is largely due to the possession of broad-spectrum beta-lactamases. The magnitude of the latter resistance has increased dramatically in some centres.

Drug-Resistant Tuberculosis

At the best of times, tuberculosis (due to *M. tuberculosis*) is a difficult infection to treat, since the bacterium is able to resist immune cells and since it is able to sequester itself in privileged body compartments. Prolonged therapy with multiple agents (which are relatively unique to the treatment of tuberculosis) has been longstanding. Over the last two decades, however, isolates of *M. tuberculosis* have emerged which are resistant to one or more of the standard anti-tuberculosis agents. This has caused concern because there are few good anti-tuberculosis agents, and the ones which are reserved as second- or third- line therapy have greater potential toxicity. The emergence of drug resistant tuberculosis has occurred for a variety of reasons, some of which include compliance problems among patients, disease in immunocompromised individuals, and use of inadequate regimens. Although drug resistant tuberculosis is recognized world-wide, many regions see it as a rarity. Tuberculosis can be a chronic illness which potentially affects any body space (although typically pulmonary). It is contagious and generally does not spare any individual.

Food For Thought

1. How does antimicrobial resistance emerge?
2. How does good infection control practice impact on the emergence of antimicrobial resistance?
3. How many antibiotic prescriptions can you recall receiving, and what have their indications been? Did you finish the prescriptions?

4. How much antibiotic is used globally? How does this total subcategorize into human and veterinary use?

Supplemental Reading

Borrell S, Gagneux S. Strain diversity, epistasis and the evolution of drug resistance in *Mycobacterium tuberculosis*. *Clinical Microbiology and Infection* Vol.17: pages 815-820 (2011).
- a good example of the dilemma that we find ourselves in

Cornaglia G, Giamarellou H, Rossolini GM. Metallo-β-lactamases: a last frontier for β-lactams? *Lancet Infectious Diseases* Vol. 11: pages 381-393 (2011).
- truth or dare?

Davis MF, Price LB, Liu CM, Silbergeld EK. An ecological perspective on U.S. industrial poultry production: the role of anthropogenic ecosystems on the emergence of drug-resistant bacteria from agricultural environments. *Current Opinion in Microbiology* Vol. 14: pages 244-250 (2011).
- how our global system of antibiotic use comes back to bite us

Enzler MJ, Berbari E, Osmon DR. Antimicrobial prophylaxis in adults. *Mayo Clinic Proceedings*. Vol. 86: pages 686-701 (2011).
- an overview of how antibiotic use may be for prevention rather than treatment

Grayson ML - ed. *Kucers' The Use of Antibiotics*. 6th Edn. Washington, DC:American Society for Microbiology, 2010.
- an extensive encyclopedic text on antimicrobials

Grundmann H, Klugman KP, Walsh T, et al. A framework for global surveillance of antibiotic resistance. *Drug Resistance Update* Vol. 14: pages 79-87 (2011).
- again a global perspective

Hicks LA, Chien YW, Taylor TH Jr, and the Active Bacterial Core Surveillance Team Outpatient antibiotic prescribing and nonsusceptible *Streptococcus pneumoniae* in the United States, 1996-2003. *Clinical Infectious Diseases* Vol. 53: pages 631-639 (2011).
- a good example of the correlation between use and evolving resistance

Lorian V - ed. *Antibiotics in Laboratory Medicine*. 5th Edition. Philadelphia, PA: Lippincott Williams & Wilkins, 2005.
- more for the enthusiast

Morgan DJ, Okeke IN, Laxminarayan R, Perencevich EN, Weisenberg S. Non-prescription antimicrobial use worldwide: a systematic review. *Lancet Infectious Diseases* Vol. 11: pages 692-701 (2011).
- a major public health dilemma of non-prescription use of antibiotics

Septimus EJ, Owens RC Jr. Need and potential of antimicrobial stewardship in community hospitals. *Clinical Infectious Diseases* Vol. 53 Supplement 1: pages 8-14 (2011)
- good antibiotic use needs to start at home and where else but our general hospitals

"For the world, I count it not an inn, but an
hospital, and a place not to live, but to die in."
Sir Thomas Browne
Religio Medici, 1642

X. Acute Care

Structure and Function

Acute care facilities are configured in many sizes and with a diversity of functions. Accordingly, the **Infection Control Service** must be tailored to meet the needs of the institution. Whereas large-sized hospitals may have meticulous infection control services, especially in a context of complex multi-specialty care, various strata of services are applicable to all acute care settings. It is tempting to generalize that a particular amount of service is required for a given number of beds, and such an accounting formula is often used by bureaucrats in hospitals. Rather, the determination of quantity of requisite service should be influenced by the real need. The nature of the acute care facility, the variety of patients that it serves, and the existing problems it faces all factor into the Infection Control Service needs.

Infection control is for everyone! The Infection Control Service of an acute care facility has many obligations, but fundamentally, it is every health care worker, and for that matter health facility entrant, that is accountable for the outcome and quality of practice. From the perspective of an organizational framework, infection control is 'managed' by an Infection Control Service, but is implemented by all. The Infection Control Service may constitute a team of individuals, a single individual, or a part-time position. The Service should not be a bureaucratic instrument but rather an applied science and practice with the ultimate goal of protecting patient, health care worker, and public. Components of the Service may be viewed as having general requirements, nursing requirements, and medical requirements. From the perspective of day-to-day practice that is tangible, most come to the realization that nursing practice is the largest subset. For hospitals of a medium to large size, the Service or team will often include an infection control officer, or medical delegate, and infection control practitioners who are most often nurses, although possibly some other health care workers who have a sufficient knowledge base that is relevant.

Figures 1 a and b. Sample reporting relationships for infection control in a large health care setting.

a.
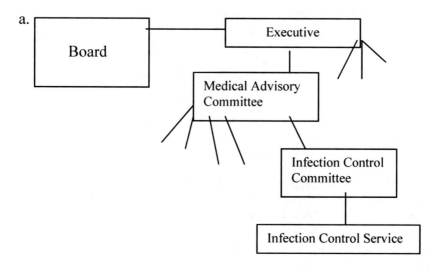

b.
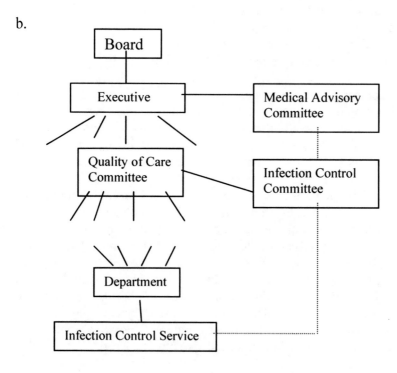

Reporting relationships of the Infection Control Service vary from institution to institution. Within the Service itself, there may be a reporting hierarchy which allows for delegation of medical and non-medical functions. The Service as a whole may then have formal reporting relationships in one or more directions. These may include medical departments or their divisions, hospital administration, risk management or quality promotion committees, medical advisory committees, among others. In most medium to large size hospitals, there is usually an **Infection Control Committee** to report to as well. Figures 1a and b demonstrate examples of possible reporting relationships in a large hospital framework.

The Infection Control Committee of an acute care facility is usually a policy-making body of individuals. Whereas this committee largely is one for policy-making in this area, it is the role of the Infection Control Service and others as detailed above to implement these policies. The size and representation of the Committee is a function of the complexity of the health care setting. Apart from representation by the Infection Control Service, it is desirable to have representation from a wide cross-section of the institution and particularly to include those areas that are mostly impacted (e.g., acute care services at high risk, nursing, employee health, sterile supply). In addition, it is of much value to be inclusive of individuals who are at the practical forefront of policy implementation including those who might be best informed to achieve the desirable outcomes of good infection control. For example, an Infection Control Committee in a pediatric hospital would benefit by including a representative of the admitting general pediatric medical staff since a large proportion of routine hospital admissions in this context are due to infections of some type. A medium-sized general hospital would benefit by representation from general practitioners who admit patients to the facility rather than having duplication by inclusion of more than one specialty internist. At the nursing level, it is desirable to include a representative who functions in the line of primary care rather than overly or solely including administrative nurses.

An **Infection Control Manual** should be prepared and made available. This Manual effectively outlines institutional policy, and it should be intended to provide a reasonably general outline and then sufficiently supportive detail in order to understand and then effectively implement practical infection control technique. The Manual should be accessible. It may not be 'everything to everyone', and it is the role of the Infection Control Service to provide supplementary interpretation or ad hoc decision-making as appropriate and required. There may be very good reason for institutional differences in certain aspects of policy and procedure, and thus, the health care professional must be conversant with the specific needs of their health care facility.

Infection Control Service Activities

The potential duties of an Infection Control Service are many, and indeed the expectations of such duties, if taken to the extreme, may be very difficult to fulfill given limitations of personnel and other resources. The needs as well as the resources of the acute care facility will dictate the emphases that an Infection Control Service should have.

In order to assist in appreciating the needs of an institution, the Infection Control Service must conduct a surveillance of the activities which relate to infection control. The surveillance can be comprehensive (i.e., including most of not all areas) or targeted and specific. It may or may not be inclusive of a mechanism to examine infection control issues both nosocomial or after hospital discharge. The intent of this surveillance is to review patient care areas, laboratory data, among other things. This may be accomplished by discussion with other staff, chart review, active observation, and follow-up. The desired outcome of understanding the norm, evaluating practice and compliance, determining the occurrence of outbreaks, and generally understanding the 'big picture' is to actually decrease or eliminate the occurrence of nosocomial infections and to provide an acceptable environment for patient care. Some of this surveillance may be passive. That is, a reporting system may be entrenched where documentation of nosocomial infections occurs by the submission of reports from front-line health care workers. Alternatively, there may be other mechanisms whereby information regarding infection control is acquired retrospectively. 'Passive surveillance' may be quite appropriate in some contexts especially when the infection control work-load is minor and the problems are few. On the other hand, some facilities will be more suited to support an 'active surveillance' program which proactively acquires, analyzes, and acts on data. The latter requires almost day-to-day vigilance in reviewing active care areas. Active surveillance is more critical for highly dynamic acute care facilities where the consequences of nosocomial infection are potentially onerous and where a considerable burden of patients with infection, and hence possible subsequent transmission, are cared for. Almost all acute health care settings maintain components of both passive and active surveillance, and the balance of emphasis is then determined by the actual needs. A tertiary referral hospital with five hundred active beds should be supported by a dedicated full-time team of health care workers who embody the Service. The Service would be proactive in surveillance and prevention for the most part but might engage in passive surveillance for some items (e.g., ongoing tally and review of clean surgical infections of which the incidence has been consistently low). If the acute care facility is a day care surgery facility, the surveillance may constitute mainly a retrospective review of post-surgical infections as determined by out-patient follow-up. Whereas the general surveillance most likely impacts on anecdotal occurrences of nosocomial or other infections in this context, the Service needs to recognize when an outbreak occurs since more obvious and widely applicable infractions may be taking place. We have previously defined 'outbreak' (Chapter V) but must re-emphasize that the actual numbers of infections which constitute an outbreak may be few if the norm is to have much fewer or none. Table 1 outlines some basic features of outbreak investigation.

The collection of data was at one time more consuming of resources given the manual nature of collection and tabulation. Computerization with its data processing capabilities of spreadsheets and databases has revolutionized this area, although one must nevertheless resign oneself to the fact that some hands-on requirements remain. Despite the availability of computerization, it may also be that the expectations and excessive detail for surveillance and analysis can overwhelm the Service (i.e., big begets bigger). It is critical therefore that the work in this area be tailored to the actual and relevant needs. It is of little value that large volumes of statistics be generated for the sake of completeness.

In addition to the aforementioned, there are a large number of potential and valuable activities that an Infection Control Service may be responsible for, if not only participate in. Again, the degree of activity in each or any of these must fit with the priority of needs, but it is easy to acknowledge that the interactions include many service areas both in and outside of the institution (Table 2).

Table 1. Components of outbreak investigation.

A. Defining a case.

B. Recognizing what has happened. Is it an outbreak?

C. Analysis of the outbreak setting.

D. Generating a hypothesis with respect to foci or causation.

E. Choosing and implementing control measures.

F. Assessment of whether control measures are beneficial.

G. Drawing conclusions and formulating preventative measures.

Table 2. A synopsis of core infection control activities.

- surveillance – active, passive or both
- data collection
- define the necessary requirements for quarantine (e.g., rooms, garb)
- design the Infection Control Manual
- participate in the Infection Control Committee
- participate in relevant standards and quality care committees (e.g., quality of care, e.g., antimicrobial use)
- stress the importance of handwashing
- education – initiation of employment and continuous
- liaison with laboratory services especially microbiology
- liaison with public health
- liaison with employee health especially with a view to monitor occupational illnesses and hazards
- liaison with the sterile supply service
- monitor hospital asepsis, disinfection, and sterilization processes
- liaison with housekeeping/janitorial services, laundry, and food services
- medical waste management

Common Problems in Acute Care

Although much of the work in Infection Control may relate to the activities as detailed in Table 2, the following illustrates the problems from a more clinical perspective. Acute care facilities by nature mostly deal with acute illnesses or needs. Given the changes in health care funding over the last several decades, acute care facilities are more likely to be dealing with more advanced and complicated illnesses. There is an increasing trend towards caring for patients with immune compromise and other (often multiple) risk factors for infection. The use of interventions and procedures and their complexity have increased considerably. The opportunity for complicated at-risk patients to contact other patients has increased, and likewise, the number of contacts with various physicians or health care workers has increased.

Infections related to intravenous devices are a major on-going problem whether for peripheral venous or central vascular access. Prevention of intravascular catheter-related infections must command a high priority in acute care. Care-givers who insert and maintain these devices must have sufficient experience and should be capable of choosing an appropriate site for insertion, select an appropriate size and type, set up the relevant associated infusate and infusion paraphernalia, and be capable of using the correct infection control precautions during the entire procedure. Replacement of the intravenous, administration sets, and infusates, as well as the appropriate maintenance of the catheter site should be expected as well.

Other foreign materials also attract infection. Infection relating to the urinary tract, respiratory tract, gastrointestinal tract, and surgical site are common place. Risk is amplified in intensive care units and burn units. The proximity of patients and the aforementioned other risks have led to the emergence of coagulase-negative staphylococci and multi-antibiotic resistant Gram negative bacteria as more common forces to reckon with. Institutional care also brings with it the special problems of infections due to agents such as *Legionella* and fungi. Due recognition must be given to the potential for hazardous encounters with needles and other sharp objects, and an injury prevention program in this regard (e.g., to implement such approaches as safe disposal of 'sharps' in puncture resistant and leak-proof containers) should be facilitated, even though it may not be the direct responsibility of infection control. Evidently, by complicating life with advanced medical care, we have also shifted the type and frequency of consequential infections.

Acute care institutions will have the burden of complicated patients who are susceptible to infection. There are many extra-ordinary issues which come of concern (Table 3). Many tailor-made approaches must be fine-tuned to accommodate such special patient care confines.

Table 3. Niche topics for special consideration during infection control planning and operations in acute care.

   A. Water supplies - re: intestinal infections, *Legionella* infection
   B. Sinks - number and positioning for adequate handwashing
   C. Showers/water aerosols - *Legionella* infection
   D. Food - *Listeria*, general food-borne pathogens
   E. New building design and renovations - inclusive of infection control concerns
       including adequate provision for isolation rooms
   F. Minimizing patient care-associated paraphernalia and clutter
   G. Laundry handling
   H. Pharmaceutical preparation, storage, and handling
   I. Pet visitation/therapy
   J. Safety of resuscitation equipment
   K. Waste management - in all of its aspects

Food For Thought

1. What roles are there for an Infection Control Service in contrast to an Infection Control Committee?
2. Review the Infection Control Manual of your health care facility.
3. An outbreak of antibiotic-resistant *Escherichia coli* urinary tract infections has occurred among the inhabitants of an auxiliary wing of a hospital. How do you approach the outbreak investigation?
4. What strategies are of value to reduce intravenous-associated infections?

Supplemental Reading

Committee on Infectious Diseases. *2009 Red Book: Report of the Committee on Infectious Diseases*. 28th Edition. Elk Grove, Ill.:American Academy of Pediatrics, 2009.
- essentially an infection control text with a pediatric focus

Fraise AP, Bradley C. *Ayliffe's Control of Healthcare-Associated Infection: A Practical Handbook*. 5th Edition. London, UK:Hodder Arnold, 2009.
- a useful handbook surviving several editions

Jarvis WR - ed. *Bennett and Brachman's Hospital Infections*. 5th Edition. Philadelphia, PA:Lippincott-Raven Publishers, 2007.
- considerably detailed and of relevance to hospitals

Mayhall CG – ed. *Hospital Epidemiology and Infection Control*. 4th Edition. Philadelphia, PA:Lippincott Williams and Wilkins, 2011.
- a voluminous text with great detail for acute care institutions

Wenzel RP – ed. *Prevention and Control of Nosocomial Infections*. 4th Edition. Philadelphia, PA:Lippincott Williams & Wilkins, 2003.
- again a voluminous text with plenty of information

"How many desolate creatures on the earth
Have learnt the simple dues of fellowship
And social comfort, in a hospital."
                    Elizabeth Barrett Browning
                    Aurone Leigh, 1857

XI. Long-Term Care

Context

Although long-term care to many implies a 'nursing home', indeed many forms of long-term care facilities are in existence. Traditional nursing homes deal mainly with geriatric populations. In addition, however, the facility may be a rehabilitation facility, pediatric chronic care setting, chronic psychiatric institute, large foster care building, palliative care environment, among others. Most work in this area is associated with geriatric residential homes, and the needs are increasing to some as many societies experience an increase in aging populations. All of these settings may have their own emphases in the area of infection control, but there are also many commonalities. The length of stay in such facilities is variable, but most are sources for transfer back to acute care since patient compromise of some sort, which leads to chronic care, is a risk factor for return to acute care. Given the increasing infection control problems in acute care facilities, a pattern of admission from and discharge to chronic care facilities serves to act as a frequent mechanism for the entry of acute care issues; both settings may act as a reservoir for the other and, in a sense, create a vicious cycle of unending inter-institutional infection. The latter is most commonly seen with multi-resistant organisms such as MRSA.

It is tempting to simply extrapolate the management of acute care infection control issues into those for long-term care, but there are many practical limitations that must be overcome or at least acknowledged. Isolation facilities for appropriate quarantine are much less likely available, and single isolation rooms may be lacking. Contact Isolation can usually be accommodated, but transfer to an acute care facility may be required for illnesses such as acute tuberculosis when Respiratory Isolation is required. Long-term care buildings are often built with little consideration, if any, for infection control needs. An 'infection control friendly' environment must certainly include strategic placement of handwashing areas. Other physical resources for infection control such as gloves, gowns, and masks may be less available, since quarantine for any infection may be much less frequently encountered.

The nature and training of care-givers in long-term care are more catered to the management of common needs. As a consequence of their background or perhaps even the milieu, acute infection control issues may not be dealt with as expeditiously or accurately as in acute care facilities. In the current era of health care restraint, long-term care areas are particularly more likely to be understaffed given the perception that most problems are not related to an acute illness. The degree of understaffing becomes more apparent when the enhanced requirements for infection control (e.g., during an outbreak) tax the understaffed care-givers even more. The nature of care in long-term facilities necessitates less physician input, and accordingly, more acute illnesses may not be as quickly attended to.

Clinical illnesses may be difficult to assess among patients of long-term care settings, and thus the recognition of an important infection may be delayed or initially missed altogether. For example, tuberculosis among the elderly may be quite cryptic in its presentation. Diagnostic facilities are most often located at a distant site, and the collection of specimens for diagnostic purposes may be less often considered perhaps due to the subsequent delayed reporting of results. The long-term care setting may find it more cumbersome to collect and transport specimens, and patients may require transfer for simple investigations such as chest x-rays.

Common Problems and Risk Factors

It has been estimated that approximately 1-15 infections occur per 1000 resident days for those who reside in nursing homes. The lower end of this frequency is consistent with usual community and family living, whereas the higher frequency exceeds the norm for most individuals in society. The simple fact of clustering individuals in a long-term care unit is in itself a risk factor for epidemic spread of infections.

Most infections among long-term care inhabitants are of the skin, respiratory tract, urinary tract, or gastrointestinal tract. Bacteremias occur as a consequence of the latter. More unique problems include pressure sores (decubitus ulcers), influenza and other viral respiratory infections, catheter-associated urinary tract infections, antibiotic-associated diarrhea, food poisoning (various forms), infection and colonization with drug-resistant bacteria (e.g., MRSA, VRE, multi-resistant coliforms), scabies, and lice. Antibiotic resistance is especially likely to occur when urinary tract infections and decubitus ulcers are being treated.

The frequency of infections, their severity, and the spectrum of infection type is highly influenced by the nature of the resident patient population. These patients may lack febrile responses and are more likely to respond poorly to treatment. Wound healing is often compromised, and there is an increased frequency of adverse reactions to treatment. Other risk factors for infection include aging and its associated changes in physiology, immobility, waning immunity, nutritional compromise, underlying illnesses (e.g., diabetes, neurological, chronic lung disease, urological dysfunction), impaired mental status, urinary or fecal incontinence, polypharmacy (including antibiotic over-use), gastric reflux and aspiration, presence of medical interventions (such as urinary catheters, intravenous lines, feeding tubes, and tracheostomies), more interaction with pets, among others. The presence of multiple risk factors is quite common.

Needs

Most if not all long-term settings should have an infection control program of some sort. What may initially be difficult to grapple with is the decision of what compromises there may be between the issues of comfort and convenience for the individual(s), and the infection control needs for the facility. Given that many long-term care facilities are viewed more as residential homes rather than health care institutions, it may seem to some as overly imposing when strict infection control practices are being proposed. The issue of risk management rather than absolute prevention becomes much more of a discussion point. In making the latter judgement, it is important to accept that some standards may be mandated by law in particular jurisdictions (e.g., federal or regional regulations). Nevertheless, a highly bureaucratic infection control program is not likely to suit a long-term care facility when resources are stretched over other issues.

A reasonable infection control program in long-term care should have several elements more or less. There should be a surveillance system which can detect problems and implement solutions. Policy and procedure should be consistent with good infection control practice. Employee education and employee health should be favourably impacted. Links with public health authorities are important. Programs for immunization (especially for influenza and *S. pneumoniae*), antibiotic use review and control, and tuberculosis surveillance may be relevant. An understanding of Standard Precautions or the equivalent should be implicit.

The infection control program in long-term care should be accountable. An Infection Control Committee should be formed. The individual(s) who function as practitioners of infection control may be designated nurses who function mainly in other capacities, but whose time is partly spared for infection control in the absence of competing interests.

There are increasing trends towards early discharge from acute care facilities and towards the caring of more complex patients in long-term care. Thus, it is imperative that good communications be had between the acute and long-term care areas. Policies relating to infection control are useful to facilitate acceptance and transfer of individuals.

Food For Thought

1. Interact with long-term care facilities in your locale. What Infection Control programs are in existence?
2. Outline major differences that you might anticipate between acute and long-term care facilities.
3. What practical considerations are there to reduce the frequency of urinary catheter-related infections?
4. What practical considerations are there to reduce the frequency of bed sores and related infections?
5. How do you manage respiratory infection outbreaks (including influenza) in long-term care facilities?

Supplemental Reading

Friedman C, et al. Requirements for infrastructure and essential infection control and epidemiology in out-of-hospital settings: a consensus panel report. *Infection Control and Hospital Epidemiology* Vol. 20: pages 695-705 (1999).
- a consensus panel report worth reading

Garibaldi RA. Residential care and the elderly: the burden of infection. *Journal of Hospital Infection* Vol. 43 (Supplement): pages 9-18 (1999).
- an excellent review with reference to the elderly

Greig JD, Lee MB. Enteric outbreaks in long-term care facilities and recommendations for prevention: a review. *Epidemiology and Infection* Vol. 137: pages 145-155 (2009).
- an example of a problematic infection for such facilities

Harris JA. Infection control in pediatric extended care facilities. *Infection Control and Hospital Epidemiology* Vol. 27: pages 598-603 (2006).
- nevertheless a long-term care facility

Smith PW, Bennett G, Bradley S, and SHEA and APIC. SHEA/APIC guideline: infection prevention and control in the long-term care facility. *American Journal of Infection Control* Vol. 36: pages 504-535 (2008).
- guidelines with broadranging concensus

Stevenson KB, Loeb M. Performance improvement in the long-term care setting: building on the foundation of infection control. *Infection Control and Hospital Epidemiology* Vol. 25: pages 72-79 (2004).
- how do we get better?

Strausbaugh LJ, Crossley KB, Nurse BA, Thrupp LD. Antimicrobial resistance in long-term care facilities. *Infection Control and Hospital Epidemiology* Vol. 17: pages 129-140 (1996).
- review this in the context of Chapter IX as well; it is no less pertinent today

Yoshikawa TT, Ouslander JG - eds. *Infection Management for Geriatrics in Long-Term Care Facilities*. 2nd Edition. New York, NY:Informa Healthcare USA, Inc., 2007.
- a general guide to infections in such facilities

"The whole earth is our hospital,
Endowed by the ruined millionaire."
Thomas Stearns Eliot
Four Quartets. East Coker, II., 1940

XII. Ambulatory, Office, and Home Care

Ambulatory Care

There may be several forms of so-called ambulatory care, but we use the term here to describe a range of services that are provided to patients who are mobile or who can be more easily and regularly transported. These services are mostly provided in clinics or centres that are affiliated with acute care institutions. Perhaps these may be regarded as more complicated forms of office practice and indeed are often associated with the latter. Common examples include attendance for out-patient infusion therapy (e.g., antibiotic or chemotherapy), endoscopy suites (e.g., gastrointestinal or respiratory), renal dialysis (mainly hemodialysis), and out-patient surgery. Certainly in the area of out-patient surgery, or day surgery, there have been considerable changes in technology which have facilitated the performance of interventions which previously could only be seen as in-patient surgery.

The needs and emphases in infection control are more similar to those which are detailed under Office Care (below), but given the nature of the more complex clinical issues, there are several additional issues which carry over from the acute care setting. Ambulatory care most often encompasses a day therapy or investigation. Visits often last for several hours. A patient may attend several different diagnostic and treatment areas during the visit, and thus the attendance to infection control concerns can be sometimes problematic if precautions are required. These care areas have a high through-put of patients compared to in-patient facilities. Medical care is more fluid and transitory; attention is increasingly given to moving the patient in an efficient manner with less concern being given to infection control matters which are by nature less of the overall care needs.

An 'entry check' for infection control-related issues should be considered especially when there is a high probability that more complex patients are likely to attend ambulatory care and may suffer more from the spread of infection. This screening at the point of admission should ask relevant questions about common and active infections. Ambulatory care areas should be required. For day surgical facilities, most infections will occur after a patient has been discharged from the ambulatory surgical centre, and most of these infections will be simple wound infections. Patient and clinic follow-up oriented reporting of these is feasible.

Office Care

Patient care in the office setting is analogous to ambulatory care as detailed above, but it takes place in more widespread and less complicated areas. These will include physicians' offices, physiotherapy and physical rehabilitation suites, distance nursing centers, alcohol and drug rehabilitation areas, among many other others. The basic infection control needs are generally the same but again, like ambulatory care, there is considerably more patient traffic. In primary care, as conducted by a general or family practitioner, a significantly large proportion of office visits relates to patients who have common infections, especially those of the respiratory tract. Daily encounters with infections are inevitable especially those of the respiratory tract. Daily encounters with infections are inevitable especially when the number of clinic visits may tally in the dozens. Since the patient population has less in the way of underlying chronic illnesses that may be considerably impacted by an acquired infection, proportionately much less attention is directed towards infection control issues when compared to acute care settings, and realistically, the nature of the infection control problem is more routine and simple (e.g., attending to the patient with a severe cold or sore throat rather than an infection with a multi-resistant bacterium).

By nature of the frequent patient contacts and common presentation of especially viral illnesses, handwashing is a critical practice. Handwashing should be considered of value both before and after patient contact or contact with potentially soiled items. Handwashing is also recommended before and after the conduct of invasive procedures, and between separate procedures although being conducted on the same patient. Other occasions for handwashing in the office include post-washroom use, after glove removal (despite the acknowledgement that the bearing of gloves in itself is protective), and when the hands are otherwise soiled during the course of other events. The basic philosophies of Standard Precautions (see Chapters VI and VII) are to be followed. The safe handling of needles and sharps in the office is also critical.

The choice of soaps for handwashing in office care has been the subject for healthy debate. Most common soaps facilitate the mechanical removal of debris, including germs, from the hands, but effective germicidal activity often warrants the use of more active handwashing agents. Given the higher frequency of encounter with infectious microbes, it would seem prudent to use the more active agents (see Chapter VIII) for both staff and patient wash areas. Alcohol rubs are increasingly popular and made available to both patient and healthcare worker.

Appropriate cleaning of inanimate objects is also of concern in office care. Simple paraphernalia such as stethoscopes, otoscopes, blood pressure monitors, scales, etc. are all subject to frequent use. Toys in the waiting areas as well as table surfaces are all subject to frequent contacts. The use of disposable supplies has helped in this area. Disinfection and sterilization are knowledge areas that must be understood by the professional staff. There should be some reasonable understanding of agents that are used for the latter since some may be especially caustic (e.g., glutaraldehyde), and others may be harmful to some materials (e.g., bleach and particular metals). Table 1 outlines some of the common office instruments or surfaces that warrant special attention. Office settings uncommonly house small autoclaves, but effective sterilization (excepting absolute spore eradication) may be achieved by boiling for 20 minutes for most objects that are heat resistant and especially those that are not used for invasive transcutaneous procedures. The processes as recommended in Table 1 reflect an assumption that sufficient resources are available for these needs. In less affluent societies, resource allocation which is comparable to 'Western' expectations may be totally impractical. The efficacy of boiling in water for those tools that withstand such treatment may well be tolerated and indeed highly efficacious for most circumstances including surgical instruments.

The use of multi-dose vials should be reduced to a minimum especially if the uses are separated by many day intervals. Multi-use eye products are particularly a hazard for transmission of viral agents that cause epidemic conjunctivitis. Carpeted floors are not recommended due to the potential for soilage. Decisions are needed in the handling of hazardous waste. Material such as tissue, blood, soiled dressings, and body fluids can be considered as biohazardous waste as may sharps containers. Urine, feces, and vaginal tampons are disposed by usual processes. Health care workers should be appropriately immunized; they should be up-to-date with routine vaccines, and they should be candidates for vaccination against hepatitis B, influenza, and chicken pox.

Illnesses with greater concern for respiratory spread (e.g., chicken pox, tuberculosis, measles) should be dealt with and prioritized efficiently, since proper air handling units are not available in office practice. If such illnesses are suspected before the office visit, it may be best to schedule the visit towards the end of the day. Since the diagnoses, however, are not often considered

Table 1. Recommended methods for decontamination of office materials and instruments.

Item	Process	Rationale
Work surfaces, baby scales, floors	Phenolic or quaternary ammonium compound or equivalent	Need low level or intermediate level decontamination for non-critical items. A 1:10 dilution of household bleach may be used specifically for blood and body fluid spills.
Stethoscopes	Isopropyl alcohol wipe	Non-critical items of frequent use
Needles and syringes, respiratory , flow meter mouthpieces	Consider disposal	
Thermometers	Consider disposable covers	Old version glass may be decontaminated
Otoscope	Isopropyl alcohol wipe of surface; immersion in 60-90% alcohol of reusable pieces	Otoscope handles and battery pack cannot be immersed. Patient contact materials require more consistent decontamination.
Non-complex metal instruments (e.g., nasal speculum, vaginal speculum, rigid sigmoidoscope, or anal speculum)	Boiling in water	Highly effective and simple; use of instrument on mucosal surfaces; not for invasive surgery; high level disinfection is desirable.
Flexible endoscopes	Initial cleaning; immersion in 2% glutaraldehyde for 20 min.	High level disinfection desirable
Surgical instruments	Heat sterilization	Sterilization desirable

beforehand, the office visit should make use of a room with a closed door, and patient entry and discharge should be expedited.

The primary physician has a role in educating the patient and family in regards to the reduction of risk for spreading infection in the home. More complicated follow-up in this regard or the need to monitor quarantine in the community largely is the responsibility of public health authorities. Community outbreaks are also under the mandate of public health authorities.

Home Care

Realignments in health care funding and the associated spin-offs have affected health care world-wide. This movement has shifted a considerable portion of hospital care to ambulatory clinics and to the home. Although there may be rightful criticisms aimed at the rapidity, nature, and necessity of such change, most will agree that a proportion of it is quite justified. The provision of home care is not a new concept, but the emphasis on home care has been emerging particularly since the 1990s. This trend has led to the presence of more complicated patients in the home, and this change has prompted the need to heighten health care standards in this context, including infection control.

Who delivers home care? The providers include home care nurses acting independently or through health care agencies. Some of these agencies are intimately linked with or are the same as large health care organizations that also provide acute care. This care may be intermittent (e.g., hourly versus day shift versus complete home co-residence). It may provide care that is not strictly medical, such as food services, hygiene, and companionship. It may relate to acute, chronic, or palliative care needs. Other critical providers of home care include the patients themselves or their family and friends.

What does home care aim to achieve? Ultimately the aim is to reduce in-hospital acute care facility utilization and thus result in net cost savings to both patient and health care system. Many patients wish to be cared for in the comfort of home and family. Psychosocial misgivings of institutional care are avoided. New technologies and increasing societal acceptance have facilitated home care, but the infection control concerns are generally the basic ones reconsidered. Table 2 highlights some common barriers to home care and, effectively, the implementation of infection control practice in this context.

Infection control issues in home care must obviously depend on patient needs and the standard of applicable practice. Isolation precautions are generally less often required than in acute care, but several patient-oriented procedures and other needs are common in this environment. Risk factors for infection are generally the same as those with long-term care. Home intravenous therapy (administered through a spectrum of venous access devices, i.e., peripheral or central) may be required for hydration, administration of antibiotics, analgesics,

Table 2. Barriers to home care and effective infection control.

1. Language barriers
2. Other cultural barriers (e.g., acceptance)
3. Family issues and/or a lack of general peer support
4. Levels of education
5. Old age
6. Lack of basic needs including any of the following: running water, refrigeration, heating, electricity, toilet facilities
7. Possible need for self-monitoring
8. Possible need for more supervision than usual home residence

and other pharmacological agents including chemotherapy, parenteral nutrition, and clotting factors. Other provisions attend to the needs of feeding tubes (peroral or direct gastric), wound care, urinary catheterization, tracheostomies, and ventilators as well as other medical devices. The complexity of these needs has become more critical as patients with immunocompromise (e.g., HIV-infected) are increasingly representative. The home care provider must be versatile with the new age of these technologies, and appropriate use and set-up is critical to infection control.

Of the most common infection control problems, complications of intravenous therapy are prominent. In particular, needle stick injuries may occur as a consequence of recapping needles or as a consequence of lacking sharps containers (Figure 1). The use of external central venous devices, multi-lumen venous devices, and some needleless systems may pose as special risk factors for patient infection. Inconsistent availability of gloves and less than desirable infectious waste disposal are also of concern. Indeed, it is not uncommon for home care providers to bring gloves, gowns, and masks as required. Wound care may require aseptic technique, irrigation and/or change of dressings. The use of chronic indwelling catheterization should be considered a tactic of last resort, and preferably, the options of intermittent catheterization, diaper equivalent, and condom (for males) catheterization should be used. When required, the indwelling catheter should be inserted with aseptic technique. It should be secured to reduce movement, urethral trauma should be reduced, and the closed system should not be opened. The frequency for routine change of indwelling catheter is open to debate, but 2-4 weeks is generally accepted unless there are complications of leaking, damage, or frank obstruction. Respiratory suction catheters can be reused for the same patient but cleaned periodically; some of these may be relatively resistant to boiling.

Figure 1. An example of a sharps container which meets modern concerns and expectations.

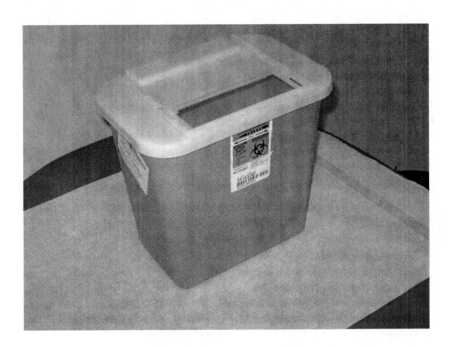

A thorough knowledge of infection control is essential for most home care providers, but it may be equally if not more important to adequately equip the patient, family, or friends with some basic knowledge, since the destiny of infection may very well be mostly in their hands. The care provider is able to instruct the patient and other home care givers in procedure and therapy. From an infection control perspective, this may include handwashing and aseptic technique, use of gloves, safe disposal of needle and biohazardous waste, and safe cleaning of the environment. Table 3 details some common indications for patients and care-givers in regard to the use of handwashing.

Several teaching points should be emphasized when sharps are a concern as highlighted in Table 4.

The diffusion of home care to many providers has certainly and greatly complicated the ability for an integrated infection control surveillance to exist in this setting. On an individual basis, reportable concerns can be addressed to the primary medical care-giver or public health authorities, but a network of

Table 3. Indications for handwashing in home care.

    A. Handling a patient with a known infection or with a reasonable infection transmission hazard.
    B. Obvious soiling of the hands.
    C. Removal of gloves
    D. Known presence of multi-resistant bacteria
    E. Between procedures
    F. Between patients
    G. Prior to invasive procedures such as urinary catheterization
    H. High risk contact with feces and urine
    I. Contact with contaminated surfaces

Table 4. Salient learning issues for home care providers whose role includes the use of sharps.

    1. Learn the technique well
    2. Refrain from recapping of needles
    3. Refrain from re-use of needles
    4. Have a safe sharps container available and dispose carefully
    5. Do not attempt to re-access materials inside of a sharps container
    6. Keep sharps containers out of the reach of children
    7. Wear gloves during sharps usage
    8. Proper disposal of sharps containers as biohazardous waste
    9. Safely clean blood spills and dispose of biohazardous waste
    10. Wash hands after glove removal
    11. Report percutaneous injuries that are required during the use of contaminated sharps

infection control practice may be feasible if a large provider of home care is responsible. As in other settings, the infection control functions could include elements of surveillance and data collection, creation of policy and procedure, education, intervention and improvement, and prevention. As the needs for organized infection control will vary greatly in this context, the following factors should weight heavily: the patient(s), underlying illnesses, nature of home care needs, demographics, presence or history of outbreaks, needs for dealing with medical waste, and occupational exposure dilemmae. Acute care facilities are often deficient in their follow-up of discharged patients especially those transferred to home care. Therefore, a feed-back loop from home care to acute care, long term care, and public health can be of value. This is of course critical in regards to outbreaks. The home care infection control program may track and tabulate infections. The data may be periodically reviewed. The infection control program can also be of benefit to the health care professional participant in regards to fast-tracking employee health issues, especially safety concerns such as needlestick injury.

The home care health professional may serve as the vector for infection as visits between homes occur. The discharge to home of patients with multi-resistant bacteria has especially made care more complicated. Home care providers also have a role to forewarn acute care and other institutions about the return or admission of home care patients who have infections. As for long-term care, the frequent movement of these patients between acute and chronic care sites and the nature of their underlying complicated illnesses increase the potential for spread of contagion.

Whether ambulatory, office, or home care, common themes emerge for consideration of special issues such as needle disposal and waste management (including diapers), storage of medicines and medical supplies, laundry, food preparation and storage, and pet exposure

Food for Thought

1. Many patients have active infections when seen in the context of ambulatory, office, and home care. Think of each of these three settings, and design a mechanism for each which allows for the screening of transmissible diseases and their quarantine in that setting.
2. When health care workers encounter patients with infections in the out-patient office, concern for transmission occurs. The likelihood of each transmission to the health care worker depends on a number of variables, but length of time for exposure is often used as the major arbiter. What length of time for exposure is considered important for:
        a) tuberculosis?
        b) whooping cough?
        c) chicken pox?
3. How should the home care provider maintain precautions for a home care patient who is known to be colonized with MRSA?

Supplemental Reading

American Academy of Pediatrics Committee on Infectious Diseases. Infection prevention and control in pediatric ambulatory settings. *Pediatrics* Vol. 20: pages 650-665 (2007).
- parallels similar concerns among other ambulatory settings

Clark P. Emergence of infection control surveillance in alternative health care settings. *Journal of Infusion Nursing* Vol. 33: pages 363-370 (2010).
- progression during changes in health care environments

Flanagan E, Chopra T, Mody L. Infection prevention in alternative health care settings. *Infectious Disease Clinics of North America* Vol. 25: pages 271-283 (2010).
- with the realization that alternative health care settings are becoming more common

Herwaldt LA, Smith SD, Carter CD. Infection control in the outpatient setting. *Infection Control and Hospital Epidemiology* Vol. 19: pages 41-74 (1998).
- an ambulatory care perspective

Jarvis WR. Infection control and changing health-care delivery systems. *Emerging Infectious Diseases* Vol. 7: pages 170-173 (2001).
- influences of massive restructuring; there will be other such cycles

Rhinehart E, McGoldrick M. *Infection Control in Home Care and Hospice.* 2nd Edition. Sudbury, MA:Jones and Bartlett Publishers, 2006.
- a detailed overview

Rice R. Infection control in the home. *Geriatric Nursing* Vol. 19: pages 297-300 (1998).
- a cogent nursing perspective

Swanson J, Jeanes A. Infection control in the community: a pragmatic approach. *British Journal of Community Nursing* Vol. 16: pages 282-288 (2011).
- a pragmatic discussion

"We must think of our whole economics in terms
of a preventive pathology instead of a curative pathology."
Richard Buckminster Fuller (1895-1983)
No More Secondhand God

XIII. Immunization and Prevention

The practice of infection control includes many techniques which are certainly preventative in nature, and reduction of risk is a key element in risk management. Beyond these forms of prevention, the medical practices of vaccination, passive immunization, and antibiotic prophylaxis are extremely important as well. Many aspects of the latter are prescribed as a function of good medical practice or public health initiative, but infection control staff may have a role in impacting on preventative practice in several ways. In large institutions, these preventative measures are often overseen and administered by an employee health bureau. In smaller settings, the same individuals may be responsible for both topics of employee health and infection control, and likely more.

Vaccination

The history of vaccination is an amazing one, and one which has brought about hope to modern medicine. Tremendous progress in vaccination has led to the marked reduction, if not disappearance, of several important infections. For example, the implementation of active polio vaccination has led to the elimination of the disease in most continents. Where vaccination for *H. influenzae* type b is now routine, there has been a tremendous reduction in invasive pediatric infections (e.g., meningitis) due to this bacterium. Whereas newer vaccines continue to emerge, there has also been great progress towards improving the existing vaccines, some of which have been practically unmodified for several decades, and towards the reduction if not elimination of side effects. Progress is not without its challenges, however, as physicians and scientists must now grapple with more complex vaccine schedules, if not only because of the large number being administered to children alone.

What is a vaccine? A **vaccine** is a structure, however complicated or simplistic, which induces the body to generate an immune response to it so that protection towards the microbe and hence infection is the net result. The vaccine may also be referred to as an **immunogen**. There are many variations on the theme regarding the nature of immunogen structure. For example, some vaccines may be live viruses or bacteria which have been sufficiently modified in the laboratory such that they are not practically pathogenic but yet retain the property of stimulating a useful immune response. Pathogenic microbes can be inactivated by a variety of processes (e.g., heat, chemical) so that they do not cause infection but yet still retain immunity provoking structures. If specific elements of a microbe are recognized as disease-causing factors (called **virulence determinants**), a protective immunity may be raised against the microbe by using one or more of these factors in the vaccine. If the immunogen is naturally a toxin (e.g., tetanus toxin), it can be inactivated in the laboratory to yield a 'toxoid' which then serves as a safe vaccine. Thus, a vaccine could be solely a protein, a polysaccharide [i.e., long complex sugar molecule(s)], or combinations of the latter with other microbial structures. For example, the first generation of vaccines to prevent *S. pneumoniae* pneumonia were developed with the use of polysaccharide extracts from the bacterium's capsule. New *B. pertussis* vaccines (whooping cough) may have more than one virulence factor immunogen which are administered simultaneously. Vaccines may be entirely natural products such as whole microbe or extracts thereof, or they may be entirely synthetic. Given the progress in developing molecular tools, the exact details of the immunogen's constitution may be known so that an entirely artificial (in laboratory) synthesis will be possible especially when the structure is relatively small. Synthetic vaccines may also combine immunogens from different microbes. For example, the polysaccharide capsule of *H. influenzae* type b was initially used as an immunogen, but immune responses were inconsistent especially in the younger age groups that suffered most from invasive *H. influenzae* type b infections. In order to improve the immune response, the polysaccharide was chemically linked to diphtheria toxoid or tetanus toxoid. The latter are modified protein virulence factors of *C. diphtheriae* and *C. tetani* respectively and to which potent immune responses occur. This chemical combination, called a **conjugate vaccine**, (see Figure 1) then provides an enhanced immune response to the previously weak immunogen. Thus, the actual protective component of a vaccine may vary from a simple short protein to multiple complex determinants of a complete microbe.

How do vaccines work? The most important desirable outcome is protection. For some infections, protection is dependent on the development of antibodies which neutralize the active germ or at least inferfere with its function or the function of a virulence factor (e.g., toxin). This antibody response may be active at the site of contact (e.g., mucosal), or it may be active systematically, and hence ward off microbial invasion. Vaccines may also be effective by recruiting cell-mediated immune responses (see Chapter III) rather than antibody

Figure 1. Schematic drawing of a conjugate vaccine.

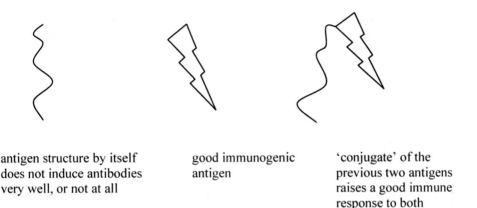

antigen structure by itself
does not induce antibodies
very well, or not at all

good immunogenic
antigen

'conjugate' of the
previous two antigens
raises a good immune
response to both
structures

production. As well, vaccines may be effective by stimulating both antibody production and cell-mediated immunity. Many vaccines have had a long history, and they were often initiated with the belief that antibody responses were the one and only factor to trigger protection. The favoured approach was presumed antibody development after inoculation by needle. When vaccines are given this way (parenteral), much of the antibody response is systemic with little or no mucosal antibody resulting. Yet, many of the pathogens that we protect against are mucosal pathogens. It is not surprising therefore that most successful vaccines (e.g., tetanus toxoid, diphtheria toxoid) protect against the effects of pathogens which cause systemic disease. Creating vaccines for mainly mucosal pathogens is much more difficult. The intended useful attributes of a good vaccine are listed in Table 1.

The need for and administration of a vaccine will depend on a number of factors. An understanding of the epidemiology of the specific infection is crucial here since the timing, population, and efforts relating to the infection will be known. Among those who suffer most from the infection, it may then be determined if a particular measure of immunity can define those who are at risk. Patients must be accessible, and the effects of immunizing some versus all should be understood. The duration of a protective immune response will vary depending on the vaccine, and such vaccination will necessarily influence the

190

Table 1. Useful attributes of a good vaccine.

      A. Provides full protection
      B. Provides long-standing immunity
      C. Is effective for all age groups
      D. Is produced easily
      E. Standardization is easy
      F. The vaccine withstands extremes of transport, storage, and use
      G. The vaccine is easily administered
      H. The vaccine is cost-effective
      I. Doe not induce any form of the infection
      J. Does not revert in any way to a virulent microbe
      K. It is free of contaminants and potentially harmful preservatives
      L. It is free of adverse effects

need for booster doses of vaccine to augment existing immunity. An understanding of vaccine complications, especially those that may be age-related, also affects the understanding of vaccine benefit versus risk of complications and the disease itself.

The spectrum of available and routine vaccines continues to increase (Table 2). Many other vaccines are available for particular needs even though their utilization is lesser (Table 3). The latter are given with a knowledge of patient demographics and risk factors. Geographic variation in vaccine administration will depend on the epidemiology of infection in that area as well as the cost. Some vaccines are mainly given to pediatric age groups, with boosters periodically administered as well.

The efficacy of vaccines is highly variable. For some vaccines, the efficacy in normal individuals approaches 100% (e.g., tetanus, diphtheria, measles) when given in a series. Repeated doses are required for many vaccines since a sizeable proportion may have inadequate responses after a single dose. Booster doses depend on the degree of waning immunity over time. In addition, some individuals do not respond well to particular vaccines. The best example of the latter is the poor response to polysaccharide vaccines among children under two years of age. Most adverse effects are mild and non-life threatening such as local pain at the site of inoculation with or without some swelling or fever. Among children, irritability and fatigue are occasionally experienced. Some of the live-attenuated viruses may cause a mild systemic illness (e.g., varicella zoster virus, rubella). Major side effects such as anaphylactic shock or central nervous system complications are generally quite rare.

Table 2. Common routine vaccines in the world. The definition of 'routine' depends on the standard in a given country.

Vaccine	Timing	Comments
diphtheria toxoid	routine childhood; boosters in adulthood	inactivated toxin
tetanus toxoid	routine childhood; boosters in adulthood	inactivated toxin
pertussis	routine in childhood	formerly inactivated whole bacterium; increasing use of component vaccines
polio	routine childhood	both live attenuated and inactivated vaccines available
pneumococcal	routine childhood	conjugate vaccine
H. influenzae type b	routine childhood	conjugate vaccine
meningococcal	routine childhood	conjugate vaccine
measles	routine childhood	live attenuated virus
mumps	routine childhood	live attenuated virus
rubella	routine childhood	live attenuated virus
hepatitis B	routine childhood	synthetic
rotavirus	routine childhood	initial vaccine was largely abandoned but new vaccines emerging
varicella-zoster virus (chicken pox)	routine childhood	live attenuated virus; not all countries are routinely immunizing

Table 3. Examples of vaccines which are in special use for high risk groups.

Vaccine	Timing	Comments
hepatitis A	high risk exposure; travelers	inactivated virus
BCG	high risk for tuberculosis (may cause positive Mantoux test)	attenuated strain of *Mycobacterium bovis*
influenza	elderly; some chronic medical conditions	inactivated virus
pneumococcal	at risk for pneumococcal pneumonia (e.g., elderly, chronic respiratory disease)	polysaccharide vaccine; conjugate vaccines
meningococcal	given in outbreak settings or in areas where disease is highly endemic	good for limited serogroups (esp. A and C); polysaccharide and conjugate vaccines
rabies	pre-exposure for high risk activity; post-exposure prophylaxis	inactivated virus
yellow fever	endemic areas (e.g., some Central American countries)	attenuated live virus
Japanese encephalitis	endemic area (e.g., SE Asia)	inactivated virus
typhoid fever	endemic areas; travelers to endemic areas	attenuated bacterium or inactivated
cholera	travelers to endemic areas	inactivated bacterium and synthetic toxin
plague	rare indications	inactivated bacterium
human papillomavirus	prevent cervical cancer in females	synthetic and conjugate vaccine
enterotoxigenic *E. coli*	travelers to endemic areas	same as for cholera

From a strictly infection control perspective, it is desirable to have staff protected against infections such as measles, mumps, and rubella for their own benefit in addition to the need to prevent secondary spread to other patients. Hepatitis B vaccination is imperative for those who are at risk for contact with blood and body fluids. The latter vaccine now has a good track record for efficacy and safety. Varicella zoster virus is currently becoming used more often in medical care areas for staff. Influenza vaccines are incompletely protective, but several reports have indicated that they may be cost-effective in reducing lost days of work. In areas of high risk for influenza epidemics (e.g., nursing homes), influenza vaccination of staff may reduce secondary spread. Effectively then, vaccines may help both employee and patients.

Passive Immunization

After acute exposure to some infections, the administration of antibody from an immune donor source may assist in prevention or the reduction of the severity of disease if it occurs. For example, a pregnant female who lacks immunity to varicella zoster virus may benefit from a **passive immunization** with varicella zoster virus immune globulin (VZIG) in order to diminish the chances of developing infection after exposure. Newborns who are exposed to hepatitis B from maternal sources at birth benefit from administration of hepatitis B immune globulin (HBIG) in addition to vaccination. This form of immunization is 'passive' in that antibody has been acquired from another source. **Active immunization** may not lead to production of antibody in a sufficiently short period of time in order to prevent disease. Immune globulins in this regard have also been used for preventing tetanus, hepatitis A, measles, and rabies.

Antibiotic Prophylaxis

For some bacterial infections, nasal colonization precedes active infection, and thus there is the possibility that the bacterium can be eradicated prior to the initiation of the illness by eliminating the bacterium with an antibiotic (see Table 4; Chapter IX). For infection control purposes, antibiotic prophylaxis may be used for contacts of patients who suffer from pertussis, invasive meningococcal disease, and diphtheria. In order for such prophylaxis to be effective, it must be given sufficiently soon after the contact. The antibiotics are often ones that have the ability to re-enter secretions after oral ingestion (e.g., rifampin).

Food For Thought

1. There are many infections which cannot be prevented by vaccines. For which of these might you want an effective vaccine? Rank the latter in order of priority.
2. Review the epidemiology of the following infections with special reference to the effect of vaccination:
    a) *H. influenzae* type b invasive infection
    b) diphtheria
    c) tetanus
    d) measles
    e) rubella
3. Hepatitis A virus is acquired by fecal-oral transmission. What is meant by fecal-oral transmission? How are family members dealt with when they are contacts of a sibling or parent who has active hepatitis A?

Supplemental Reading

Levine MM, Dougan G, Good MF, et al. - eds. *New Generation Vaccines.* 4th Edition. London, UK:Informa Healthcare, 2009.
- an enthusiast's look at pending innovation

National Center for Immunization and Respiratory Diseases. Immunization of health-care personnel. *Mortality Morbidity Weekly Report* Vol. 60(RR-07): pages 1-45 (2011).
- a detailed contemporary pattern of recommended practice

Plotkin SA, Orenstein W, Offit PA. *Vaccines: Expert Consult.* 5th Edition. Philadelphia, PA: Saunders, 2008.
- a very detailed and thorough resource

Plotkin SA - ed. *History of Vaccine Development.* New York, NY: Springer, 2011.
- a multiauthored perspective on how vaccines came to be

World Health Organization. *International Travel and Health: Vaccination Requirements and Health Advice.* Geneva: WHO Publications, 2005.
- the world is a small place

World Health Organization. *State of the World's Vaccines and Immunization.* 3rd Edition. Geneva: WHO Publications, 2009.
- a solid overview of what is internationally accepted

"Will all great Neptune's ocean wash this blood
Clean from my hand?"
>William Shakespeare
>*Macbeth* II, ii, 61

XIV. Hazards in the Workplace

Health care professionals are exposed to infectious biohazards in the workplace on a near daily basis, and the degree of risk obviously depends on the specific work profile, degree of patient contact, and likelihood of interacting with a patient who suffers from an active infection. Centuries ago, prominent physicians and anatomists refused to perform autopsies on patients who suffered from suspected tuberculosis given that there was a well-known risk of transmission to the health care worker. Such concerns or similar are no less today, and indeed the wide array of infectious agents that are of known concern for transmission has increased. Most infections acquired in the workplace are due to respiratory viruses, and it must be acknowledged that the transmission of the same from ill staff to patients is also of a concerning frequency.

Who is at risk? All health care workers may acquire the same infections in the workplace as they may in the community, but those who have more direct patient contact are at greatest risk for patient-acquired infections. In addition to acquisition through direct contact and to a lesser degree respiratory spread, the transmission of blood-borne agents (e.g., HIV, hepatitis B, hepatitis C), especially from needlestick injuries, continues to be a timely subject. Personnel who work in microbiology and virology laboratories are evidently at risk for becoming infected with the microbes that they culture if not from the specimens themselves, but such infections are quite uncommon in the modern laboratory in large part due to the knowledge these people bear regarding aseptic technique and biohazards. Other laboratory personnel are more likely to be at risk for infection from blood-borne agents especially as they handle blood products. Those who perform autopsies are at risk from blood-borne agents and tuberculosis. Surgeons and dentists as well as their direct assistants are at risk for blood-borne agents, and dentists and anaesthetists are also more likely to encounter respiratory viruses and herpes simplex virus (the latter from cold sores). Transmission of infection to laundry workers has also been documented but appears to be uncommon overall.

Whereas we can measure risk to health care workers given the details of the exposure, the implications of risk go far beyond what we can measure. Perceived risk by the health care worker can be followed by anxiety and fear. The individual may express guilt and perhaps reflect anger. Concerns regarding blood-borne pathogens may affect personal relationships when transmission to family or personal contacts is considered. The outcome of infection for the health care worker can incur sick leave and alterations in professional practice. Secondary spread to patients may also be of concern.

Standard Precautions, which are augmented with further precautions as are appropriate to the context, will prevent the transmission of the vast majority of infections from patient to health care worker. There are three deficiencies, however, which have a role in promoting health care worker illness. Firstly, failure to wash hands or inadequate washing technique have a major part. Inappropriate or complete lack of isolation technique or facilities are probably next most important. Thirdly, lack of vaccination among health care workers for common preventable diseases can allow for a susceptible pool that may participate in spreading infection during an outbreak.

Safe acquisition and transport of clinical specimens is imperative. When the latter are carried out well, the transmission of suspected as well as unsuspected pathogens is prevented. Specimens should be clinically relevant. Clean and explicit instructions for specimen collection and transport should be provided. The specimen container should be adequately labeled, and it should be one that is leak proof and reasonably damage resistant. The specimen container should be transported preferentially in a sealable plastic bag. The requisition should not be placed in the bag so to avoid soilage with a potentially leaky specimen. Local guidelines may dictate transportation conditions between institutions, and other regulations are available to indicate how such potentially dangerous goods should be handled otherwise (e.g., mail, flight, courier).

The handling of tissue specimens or even the autopsy should be conducted with the utmost of care and should essentially proceed with common standards of aseptic technique. Beyond the latter, special consideration should be given to tuberculosis (due to aerosol spread), blood-borne pathogens, and prions (Creutzfeldt-Jakob Disease).

The following issues are among those which especially have raised concern for the health care worker:

Influenza

In acute care settings, influenza is not a common nosocomial infection, and health care workers are reasonably protected when applying Standard

Precautions and more pointedly Respiratory Isolation or such similar. In chronic care facilities, however, explosive outbreaks of influenza are more likely to occur, and the consequences of outbreaks are more likely to be felt given the health compromise already in existence for inhabitants, (e.g., nursing homes). Recent evaluations of influenza vaccine efficacy indicate that some infections can be prevented, and others may be lessened in intensity, although the influenza vaccines are far from perfect. Influenza vaccine has highly been promoted for health care workers in order to prevent and reduce disease, and thus decrease the opportunity for secondary spread. The ability for influenza viruses to change from year to year will complicate vaccine use. (note: in addition to influenza, respiratory virus infection as a whole poses problems to health care workers especially given that the symptoms of many types of infection may overlap with influenza. Such concern was crystallized when the SARS outbreak of 2002-2003 appeared - see Chapter XVII)

Chickenpox

In pediatric settings, chickenpox continues to be seen, and the non-immune health care worker is at risk for acquisition of the responsible virus by direct contact or aerosol spread. The potential for aerosol transmission especially makes this infection one capable of explosive spread. Fortunately, most health care workers (usually >80-90%) are immune on the basis of previous infection. Zoster eruptions (which are late but usually well-localized recurrences of varicella-zoster virus (VZV) infection) also pose a risk for transmission by direct contact, and this form of VZV illness not uncommonly occurs in the elderly. The availability of VZV vaccine has the potential to reduce the risk for both patients in the community and health care workers. Many institutions now have active employee health policies which include the screening of staff for VZV immunity and the subsequent immunization of staff who are deemed non-immune. The vaccine is not fully protective, however, and thus some consideration may still be warranted when vaccinated individuals are exposed to live virus.

Tuberculosis

Tuberculosis is one of the most common active human infections worldwide. In well-developed countries, the frequency of tuberculosis is much less, and accordingly, the infection is sometimes not considered on a timely basis. Acquisition of infection from contact in endemic areas (i.e., travel), transmission of infection from immigrants of endemic areas, and reactivation in the elderly continue to be problematic. As well, difficulty with the treatment of those infected who are severely immunocompromised (e.g., patients with AIDS), and the emergence of *M. tuberculosis* bacteria which are resistant to commonly used anti-tuberculous agents, have complicated the management and containment of tuberculosis. Health care workers should be screened for past or active infections by skin testing (Mantoux test) at the initiation of employment and regularly (e.g., yearly) thereafter if there is sufficient risk in the workplace for tuberculosis. Patients in chronic care placement such as the elderly should also be screened since they pose risk for reactivation. Physicians must not be hesitant to investigate for tuberculosis at the earliest possible convenience if and when the illness is considered. In areas of high risk for tuberculosis, some authorities recommend the use of BCG vaccine for health care workers; this vaccine is only partially effective but apparently does significantly lower the risk for infection. When caring for patients with tuberculosis, high efficiency masks are recommended to nullify airborne spread, and this approach has become ever so necessary in areas where drug-resistant tuberculosis is encountered.

Viral Gastroenteritides

Viruses are the most common cause of infectious diarrhea in the general community. Most illnesses are generally benign and self-limited, and the worst illnesses are more likely to be seen among the very young (i.e., < 1 year of age) or the very old. The amount of virus shed in stools from infected patients is considerable, and the likelihood of secondary transmission is high. It is not uncommon to see secondary spread to staff and other patients. Strict adherence to the principles of Enteric Isolation or such similar are usually sufficient. New rotavirus vaccines are emerging.

Risks During Pregnancy

The majority of health care workers within the immediate vicinity of patients are female, and some of these individuals will function in the workplace during pregnancy. Although most infections do not pose an added risk for the pregnant health care worker, there are several exceptions. Parvovirus and rubella can both infect the pregnant female and thereafter cross the placenta to harm the fetus; the effects of fetal infection are more profound during the first trimester of pregnancy. Although appropriate precautions will prevent acquisition of these infections by the pregnant health care worker, the potential for any reasonable risk to the pregnancy has led some to recommend that pregnant health care workers should not care for patients with such infections if at all possible when they are not immune. Cytomegalovirus (CMV) poses a dilemma in this regard.

This virus is well recognized as a potential cause of fetal infection, and it may certainly be acquired from patients. CMV, however, can be acquired by the fetus from mothers who have reactivated a previous infection that is dormant. In addition, most acquisitions from patients can be prevented by adherence to Standard Precautions. Many patients asymptomatically excrete CMV in urine or saliva when well or during other illnesses, and the vast majority of these excretions are not known. Hence, the health care worker is commonly exposed to CMV unknowingly. In view of the latter facts, pregnant females have not been excluded largely from the health care workplace, although some have advocated that they may be excused from caring for patients who are known to excrete very large quantities of viruses (e.g., known congenital CMV infection in a newborn).

Creutzfeldt-Jakob Disease (CJD)

As discussed in Chapter II, this illlness is caused by the transmission of a protein (not live microbe) that is generally resistant to decontaminating agents. Usual methods of decontamination and sterilization of medical instruments may not sufficiently eliminate the protein, and modifications of standard practice must be considered. The use of disposable items during neurosurgery on these patients is encouraged. The transmission from patient to health care worker is largely theoretical here, but conceivably could include transmission during needlestick injuries from sharps that are used while performing neurosurgery or ophthalmological surgery on infected patients, or while conducting autopsies or performing pathology studies of central nervous system tissue.

Viral Hemorrhagic Fevers

These illnesses include several that are caused by viruses that lead to systemic illnesses which have a high mortality rate (e.g., Ebola or Marburg viruses). The concern for these entities has been heightened and made popular by outbreaks mainly in Africa and by the risk for importation to other countries via travel. Media attention and the film industry have also popularized these illnesses. Realistically, there is a small chance for encountering these viruses outside of endemic areas. Much transmission in endemic areas is explained by local living conditions and by the transfer from patient to care-givers (especially family) who attend to these patients but who do so while lacking precautionary measures. Strict Isolation or equivalent precautions are generally sufficient.

Hepatitis B

Diagnostic testing for hepatitis B was available several decades ago, and knowledge of patient status has some part in preventative strategies, but the availability of an effective hepatitis B vaccine has provided even more in the way of protection. Health care workers are certainly at increased risk for the acquisition of hepatitis B in the acute care setting, and the most at risk include dentists, laboratory workers, hemodialysis technicians, nurses, and physicians. The latter individuals have had 5-10 times more infection than the average population. The prevalence of hepatitis B in any given population is quite variable. Percutaneous injury represents the most common mechanism for health care worker infection. Many infections will occur asymptomatically. Whereas the infected patient is a risk for the health care worker, so too is it that the infected health care worker is a risk for patients especially when the infected health care worker may be performing invasive procedures. Other mechanisms of hepatitis B transmission are likely since not all acquisitions can be accounted for by needlestick injuries.

After a needlestick injury, the risk for transmission from patient to health care worker can vary between 1-30%. The lower end of this frequency is more likely for source blood that carries hepatitis B but that lacks a particular diagnostic marker called 'E antigen'. E antigen-positive hepatitis B carrier blood poses the much higher risk. Nevertheless, all transmissions have the potential risk for severe acute liver disease during infection. Up to 10% of these infections may lead to chronic liver disease such as cirrhosis, and a smaller percentage are at risk for hepatocellular carcinoma.

The routine vaccination of health care workers of concern has markedly changed the issue of risk. Two or three vaccinations are usually administered, and post-vaccine efficacy is well over 90% for most populations. It is believed that full vaccination in this regard is followed by long-lasting immunity, although the need for booster vaccine after many years is still a subject for healthy debate. In addition, the routine use of vaccine for the general population has been adopted in many societies. Non-immune health care workers who are exposed to blood and body fluids by way of percutaneous injury or mucosal splash should be investigated as should the blood of the source patient. Known exposures to hepatitis B should receive both hepatitis B immune globulin and vaccine.

The routine administration of hepatitis B vaccine should not lead the health care worker to complacency. Some vaccine recipients, albeit few, do not respond to the vaccine. Furthermore, whereas hepatitis B acquisition may be prevented, significant exposures still bear the risk for acquisition of hepatitis C and HIV. It is not uncommon to see patients who are co-infected with these microbes. In the past, known hepatitis B-positive carriers were isolated in hospitals with what was then termed Blood and Body Fluid Precautions. The latter terminology and approach have been abandoned because the status of most hepatitis B infected patients is unknown at the time of an incident. Hence, it is more rational to treat all patients as if they have the potential to transmit hepatitis B or other blood-borne agents – thus, the need for adherence to Standard Precautions.

Hepatitis C

The recognition of hepatitis C as an entity was established only over two decades ago. A diagnostic test became available by the early 1990s, and thereafter, there has emerged a much better understanding of the epidemiology. Prior to these discoveries, it had been accepted that transmissible hepatitis could occur that was not hepatitis B or hepatitis A (so-called non-A, non-B hepatitis). Most of the latter proved to be due to hepatitis C.

In most general populations, the prevalence of hepatitis C is $\leq 1\%$. This frequency is significantly higher among recipients of blood products prior to 1990 and among drug users. Acquisition occurs by the same mechanisms as for hepatitis B. Again, infection is more common in health care workers and especially those as detailed previously for hepatitis B. After needlestick injuries, infection with hepatitis C occurs in 1-10%. Preventionist strategies are aimed at reducing exposures. No passive or active immunization is available at this time. Fortunately, the success rate of treating hepatitis C with noval antiviral therapies is improving considerably.

Human Immunodeficiency Virus (HIV)

Occupational acquisitions of HIV infection have been reported and are of major concern given the potential outcome for the health care worker. Due regard for Standard Precautions is imperative, and the most important aspect of prevention remains those measures that reduce exposure. Both needlestick injuries and mucosal splashes provide risk to the health care worker. After such an exposure, the acquisition of HIV is 0.1-0.5%. There are several risk factors which are associated with infection after exposure and these include more penetrating injuries, obvious blood contamination with source blood, direct placement of needle into a blood vessel, a needlestick accident from a larger bore needle, and having the source patient ill with advanced illness (e.g., AIDS rather than asymptomatic HIV infection). These latter risk factors are essentially indicative of the risk being greater with an exposure to a high virus load.

The management of an exposure is outlined in Figure 1. The initial phase of the investigation simply focuses on management of the injury and the

202

Figure 1. An approach to the management of percutaneous and mucosal contacts with clinical specimens.

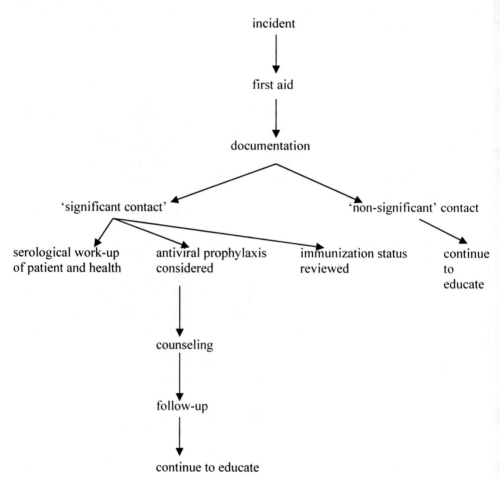

collection of blood samples from health care worker and source patient. Prior to the availability of anti-retroviral agents, no effective intervention was available. Cumulative data regarding the outcome of exposure and subsequent infection, however, have given rise to the belief that the antiretroviral agent zidovudine (AZT) may be effective for prevention when administered soon after the exposure. Such a belief evolved after an analysis of retrospective exposure data, although no formal prospective study was ever devised. Indeed, zidovudine prophylaxis is now commonly administered after high risk exposure as determined by clinical history or patient testing. The latter approach, however, was theoretically challenged given the issue of evolving HIV drug resistance. Soon after anti-viral agents were developed and clinically used for HIV infections, drug resistance emerged. AZT was essentially the first useful antiviral in this category, and therefore concern arose regarding the use of AZT alone when source patients and hence the viral infection had likely already been exposed to this drug. Current HIV therapy more often includes combinations of two or more agents. Thus, it has been recommended by many that HIV prophylaxis after exposure should include two or three agents (e.g., combinations of zidovudine, lamivudine, tenofovir, emtrictabine, didanosine, stavudine, lopinavir, among others). Countries and health agencies vary for recommendations in regards to the specific combination of preference. The use of these agents for post-exposure prophylaxis should not be taken lightly since severe adverse effects have been recorded despite the use of prophylactic agents for a short time (usually total of one month after exposure when the suspicion for infection of the source patient is confirmed or highly suspected). Antiviral use in this context is recommended very early (preferably within a few hours) after exposure, and the choice of antiviral regimen (i.e., single versus multiple) should be confirmed with the assistance of experts in the field. Follow-up for tolerance and compliance, let alone infection, is imperative. Again, there should nevertheless be great emphasis on prevention and then timely and targeted selective use of anti-retroviral agents for post-exposure prophylaxis. A clear strategy to manage all such exposures should be openly articulated and available.

Different body substances carry variant risk of HIV transmission (Table 1). Exposure to HIV and its subsequent ramifications are considerably troubling for the affected healthcare worker even when no transmission ultimately occurs - the counseling aspect that accompanies the assessment, treatment, and/or follow-up is very important.

Co-ordination

Hazards in the workplace are directly the mandate of services generally referred to as Occupational Health & Safety or Employee Health. In larger institutions, these areas are organizationally distinct from the Infection Control Service even though they are highly interactive. In small operations, however, some organizations choose to have the two functions under the same roof. These are purely matters of convenience, but the Employee Health mandate extends much beyond the issues of infection hazards in the workplace. In the least, these areas as well as the Infection Control Committee must be collaborative in developing policy and procedure which attends to the needs of diminishing the transmission of infectious agents between health care worker and patient.

A program should be in place to reduce risk, and it should have in the least all of the features as detailed in Table 2.

Table 1. Examples of low and high risk body substances for transmission of HIV. Degree of blood tainting for low risk substances may alter the ranking.

Low risk	High risk
saliva	blood
sweat and tears	tissues and organs
vomitus	body cavity fluids (e.g., peritoneal, pleural, joint)
urine	spinal fluid
stool	semen
	burn and wound exudates
	amniotic fluid

Table 2. Risk reduction for hazards in the workplace.

A. Plan a program, implement and monitor the program, and evaluate its functioning and usefulness.

B. Identify who is at risk and for what.

C. Educate on initiation of employment – stress handwashing and Standard Precautions.

E. Educate throughout employment by continuing medical education.

F. Adequately staff services.

G. Provide necessary resources including safety-oriented supplies.

H. Have an immunization program.

I. Have a program for attending to acute incidents that require attention.

J. Ensure liaison with the Infection Control Service so that health care worker exposure is minimized.

Food For Thought

1. In your professional capacity, what infectious risks have you encountered? (Think of the nature of risk and it prevention.)
2. Masks are intended to prevent acquisition of airborne germs or to prevent the patient from acquiring salivary germs from the health care worker. Outline the physics of how masks work, and then postulate what limitations there may be in currently designed masks.
3. For your health care setting, outline the processes that are in place to handle needlestick injuries.
4. What return to work schema do you propose for the healthcare worker who is suffering a likely viral respiratory infection?
5. A healthcare worker is injured with a percutaneous needle that was used to draw blood from an HIV-positive patient. The worker is afraid to receive antiviral agents. How do you counsel this person?

Supplemental Reading

Baussano I, Nunn P, Williams B, Pivetta E, Bugiani M, Scano F. Tuberculosis among health care workers. *Emerging Infectious Diseases* Vol. 17: pages 488-494 (2011).
- why we screen healthcare workers for infection

Charney W. *Handbook of Modern Hospital Safety.* 2nd Edition. Boca Raton, FL:CRC Press, Taylor and Francis Group, 2010.
- an extensive illustrated review of hazards in the workplace including those related to infectious diseases

Gabriel J. Reducing needlestick and sharps injuries among healthcare workers. *Nursing Standards* Vol. 23: pages 41-44 (2009).
- forever a concern

Hamlyn E, Easterbrook P. Occupational exposure to HIV and the use of post-exposure prophylaxis. *Occupational Medicine* Vol. 57: pages 329-336 (2007).
- a solid review

Hood J. The pregnant health care worker - an evidence-based approach to job assignment and reassignment. *AAOHN Journal* Vol. 58: pages 329-333 (2008).
- probing into a niche problem

Huber MA, Terezhalmy GT. HIV: infection control issues for oral healthcare personnel. *Journal of Contemporary Dental Practice* Vol. 8: pages 1-12 (2007).

206

- concern for all healthcare workers

Jagger J, Perry J, Gomaa A, Phillips EK. The impact of U.S. policies to protect healthcare workers from bloodborne pathogens: the critical role of safety-engineered devices. *Journal of Infection and Public Health* Vol. 1: pages 62-71 (2008).
- tools engineered for our protection

Lee R. Occupational transmission of bloodborne diseases to healthcare workers in developing countries: meeting the challenges. *Journal of Hospital Infection* Vol. 72: pages 285-291 (2009).
- an international perspective

Michelin A, Henderson DK. Infection control guidelines for prevention of health care-associated transmission of hepatitis B and C viruses. *Clinics in Liver Disease* Vol. 14: pages 119-136 (2010).
- a meticulous look at hepatitis B and C transmission

Panlilio AL, Cardo DM, Grohskopf LA, Heneine W, Ross CS. Updated U.S. public health service guidelines for the management of occupational exposures to HIV and recommendations for postexposure prophylaxis. *Mortality Morbidity Weekly Report* Vol. 54(RR09): pages 1-17 (2005).
- detailed view of American guidelines on the subject

Tarantola A, Abiteboul D, Rachline A. Infection risks following accidental exposure to blood or body fluids in health care workers: a review of pathogens transmitted in published cases. *American Journal of Infection Control* Vol. 34: pages 367-375 (2006).
- examining the published evidence

van den Berg-Dijkmeijer ML, Frings-Dresen MH, Sluiter JK. Risks and health effects in operating room personnel. *Work* Vol. 39: pages 331-344 (2011).
- a plenary view of risk including infection

Young TN, Arens FJ, Kennedy GE, Laurie JW, Rutherford G. Antiretroviral post-exposure prophylaxis for occupational exposure. *Cochrane Database of Systematic Reviews* CD002835 (2007).
- weighing the science for important decision-making

"In the discovery of secret things and in the investigation of
hidden causes, stronger reasons are obtained from sure
experiments and demonstrated arguments than from probable
conjectures and the opinions of philosophical speculators
of the common sort."

William Gilbert
De Magneta, 1600

XV. Infection Control Sleuths

Surveillance

We have detailed the many roles and concerns that comprise the activity of infection control. Whereas much of this work is active and does not require intervention as much as it does active implementation of common policy and procedure, the Infection Control Service does have an investigative role. The first phase of investigation is surveillance which essentially relates to data gathering. The second phase, if required, then leads to a scrutiny of this surveillance data which may seem to some as detective work. Most such scrutiny is but a natural consequence of the overall process. Data and observations are gathered, and they may or may not lead to hypothesis generation if the outcome is not obvious. The hypothesis is an indication of whether there is or is not a problem that may be solved, and further investigation will then more definitively review the data, possibly acquire more, and then test the hypothesis. The latter approach sounds perhaps scientific, and yet we acknowledge that most infection control dwells on behaviour and the obvious. The scientific aspects of infection control are rewarding, however, in that precision, discovery, and resulting beneficial outcomes can be measured. These scientific aspects of infection control are good reason to believe in infection control sleuths.

Fingerprinting

The gains in science have greatly impacted on infection control **epidemiology**, and in particular, there are now many methods which can be used to '**fingerprint**' micro-organisms. These methods have best been developed for bacteria. In essence, a common origin for microbes may be inferred by demonstrating that they have qualities or characterizations which are highly similar if not exactly the same. Alternatively, many differences between 'isolates' (see Chapter II) of a given species infers dissimilarity and lack of a common source. Therefore, much like the fingerprinting of humans for purposes of criminal or forensic purposes, so too microbes can often be fingerprinted in assisting the determination of common source when more than one isolate is obtained. Molecular techniques are most commonly used for this purpose, and indeed many elaborate, reliable, and helpful variations of this technology have emerged.

When are such highly investigative and scientific methods likely to be performed? In some circumstances, common sense prevails, and an outbreak may be obvious as may the causative microbe and source. Fingerprinting methods may then be of very little value. In outbreaks where commonality is less certain, such information may be crucial. Although the technology for fingerprinting has simplified tremendously, it remains that such investigations are usually the mandate of a referral centre or large laboratory. The needs are purely dictated by the complexity of the circumstances and the given needs that arise. We have previously detailed components of outbreak investigation (Table 1; Chapter X) and provided a definition of an outbreak (Chapter V). Traditionally, outbreak investigation is intended for the short-term control of infection, although certainly outbreaks can become subacute or chronic. The incidents may have occurred over a few days to several weeks or months, and the number of isolates to be studied may be as few as two to as many as the outbreak seemingly includes. The fingerprinting is essentially then a comparative study which assesses new isolates side-by-side with previously existing ones. Essentially, one determines whether there is 'clonality'; a '**clone**' is a group of a species' isolates that have significantly greater similarity than would be anticipated for randomly occurring isolates otherwise acquired, and thus the common isolates are likely derived from the same single origin. Fingerprinting can also be applied to an epidemiological surveillance which has very little to do with a focal outbreak. In the latter, there is a longer term assessment of commonality which may be applicable to geographic spread over years and perhaps to prolonged endemic activity and lengthy epidemics.

When applying fingerprinting techniques to outbreaks, it is desirable to have a method which has the features of '**typeability**' (most if not all isolates can be typed in the system), high discriminatory power (i.e., reasonably differentiates unrelated clones), reproducibility (fingerprint pattern is reproducible), and stability (fingerprint of isolates from a clone do not quickly change from patient to patient). A single fingerprinting assessment of the isolates from an outbreak may be sufficient. For the purposes of larger epidemiological surveillance, however, the method may allow for the determination of some minor changes among bacteria that occur over a longer time. Examples of fingerprinting methods have been standardized in order to allow for standard nomenclature, dispersal of methods, and comparisons among many laboratories world-wide.

Current fingerprinting techniques are based on unique features of the bacterial genome. The genetic material of bacteria includes a typical single long double-stranded DNA molecule. In addition, there may or may not be additional much smaller circular or linear double-stranded DNA molecules called plasmids. A number of elements from this genetic material may be mobile [e.g., transposons or jumping genes, insertion sequences, and bacterial viruses (bacteriophages)], and thus active change in the DNA can occur. Given this constitution, there are two major ways by which the genetic make-up of bacteria can change. Firstly, change can occur by spontaneous mutation. Secondly, there may be a transfer of genetic material between bacteria, and such transfer can occur between related and unrelated bacteria. Over time, such changes can be cumulative to the point that fundamental changes occur in the fingerprint of the bacterium. Thus, such change, which can occur during the course of active or chronic bacterial infection, during the presence of the bacterium in the environment or other reservoir, or during asymptomatic carriage among human or other living forms including animals, may affect the appreciation of commonality.

Historically, typing methods were developed on the basis of the available microbiological and biochemical tools. As detailed in Table 1, some of these methods were relatively simplistic. As advances were made in the basic sciences, more sophisticated methods were developed. In addition, the more sophisticated methods were also developed in response to the perceived inadequacies of existing tools. Overall, the trend has been towards the creation of standardized molecular methods. The latter are numerous in variation and details of their performance, and differences are not overly relevant for our discussion, but Figure 1 demonstrates an example of one such approach. Molecular methods have been simplified, and their use is now commonplace. Some of these methods are similar to the molecular techniques that are currently being used to 'fingerprint' human tissue for forensic purposes.

Fingerprinting methods have been described for essentially all of the common bacteria and they may be used for almost every outbreak imaginable. Some methods, especially molecular, are broadly applicable regardless of the bacterial species. Most applications will be targeted towards focal outbreaks, usually in hospital settings. Others will be targeted to inter-institutional outbreaks, and yet others towards outbreaks on a much larger scale. These may be applied to bacterial isolates for humans, animals, and food sources. Table 2

Figure 1. Schematic diagram of one molecular fingerprinting technique called 'pulse field gel electrophoresis' which can be used for the typing of bacterial species. DNA is isolated from the bacterium and then cut into small pieces by an enzyme. The different sizes of small DNA fragments are then resolved into a fingerprint pattern which is specific for the given strains of that species.

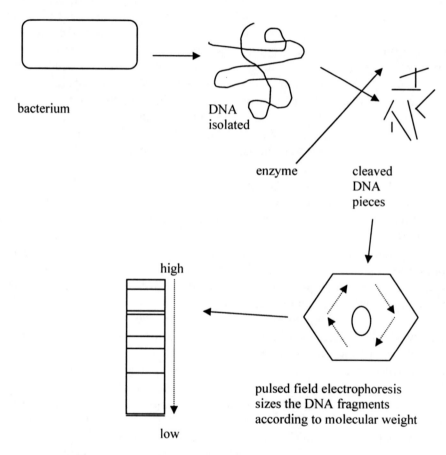

ladder pattern of DNA fragments
yields a fingerprint pattern which
is characteristic for the particular strain

Table 1. Methods for fingerprinting or typing bacteria.

Method	Mechanism
Biotyping	Exploits the variability of biochemical characters of a given species. Strains are similar when the biochemical characters are identical. This method may serve as a simple first-line approach for comparisons.
Antibiograms	Isolates of the species are deemed to be similar when their antibiotic susceptibility profiles are identical. This method may serve as a simple first-line approach for comparisons.
Serotyping	Surface structures (or antigens) of the bacterium may be variable (e.g., proteins, carbohydrates). Animals are immunized with different strains, and the post-immunization animal serum is used to react differentially with the variant bacteria.
Phage typing	Species' isolates are differentially susceptible to a series of bacterial viruses called phages.
Bacteriocin typing	Discrimination among isolates is based on their differential susceptibility to or production of natural inhibitors produced by bacteria.
Protein electrophoresis	An electrochemical method is used to show variation in sizes and distribution of proteins among isolates.
Multilocus enzyme electrophoresis	A complex method which is based on the analysis of variation among common bacterial enzymes.
Molecular methods	A wide range of tools which directly differentiates isolates on the basis of their genetic make-up. Such methods include restriction endonuclease analysis (REA), pulse field gel electrophoresis (PFGE), ribotyping, restriction fragment length polymorphism (RFLP) with nucleic acid probes, arbitrarily primed polymerase chain reaction (PCR), randomly amplified polymorphic DNA (RAPD), inter-repeat element PCR, plasmid profiling, and nucleic acid (DNA) sequencing, and microarray typing.

Table 2. Common uses for fingerprinting methods.

1. Methicillin-resistant *Staphylococcus aureus*

2. Multi-resistant coliforms in hospitals

3. *Pseudomonas*-like organisms and outbreaks involving environmental sources

4. Food-borne pathogens (e.g., *E. coli* O157:H7, *Salmonella*)

5. Vancomycin-resistant *Enterococcus* spp.

6. *Mycobacterium tuberculosis* – community epidemiology

7. *Streptococcus pneumoniae* – vaccine serotyping

outlines some common uses for fingerprinting techniques.

For fingerprinting methods that are very reproducible and which can be performed in several different laboratories, networks may be developed whereby fingerprinting is performed in regional centres, and their data is analyzed for similarity at a central location. Information arising can then be sent back to the regional centres for action if need be, and widespread outbreaks may be ascertained.

The following example illustrates the use of one molecular fingerprinting method:

During a seven day period, three cancer patients on the same ward developed a blood-borne infection due to the bacterium Stenotrophomonas maltophilia. *This bacterium is in many ways similar to* Pseudomonas aeruginosa *in that it is a common environmental organism. It causes infections practically only among patients who have complicated medical illnesses. It has historically been linked with intravenous devices and infusates. The three patients so affected had different malignancies, were being treated at very different stages of their illnesses, and were occupying separate rooms. A quick review of each circumstance revealed the following commonalities: common medical staff, common nursing staff, presence of central venous lines which required heparin infusion, receipt of multiple antibiotics, and all having daily bloodwork to assess routine blood and chemistry indices. Otherwise among the large number of cancer patients cared for by the same cancer group, S. maltophilia blood-borne infection was experienced approximately 6-12 times per year and was* numerically one of the least common blood-borne pathogens among these patients. Nevertheless, concern was voiced as to whether the cluster of three represented an outbreak or whether these infections were but simply part of the background frequency. Others expressed concern that there might be commonality for all S. maltophilia infections and that their infrequency was due to the low virulence potential for these bacteria. Isolates from the cluster, as well as those from seemingly sporadic episodes for many months prior, were subjected to a molecular typing method known as inter-repeat element PCR which is highlighted in the Figure 3. Results of this fingerprinting are shown in Figure 2. The three isolates from the clustered blood-borne infection are identical in contrast to the fingerprint patterns of those isolates from other bacteremias; the latter were all different from each other. The occurrence of an outbreak was therefore supported. Further investigation determined that a single multi-dose heparin vial was being used for all three patients; this item had been prepared by the hospital pharmacy. Culture of the heparin solution also yielded S. maltophilia which was subsequently found to be of the same fingerprint pattern. Removal of the item was followed by a lack of any further such infections. Within the next several months, however, no further S. maltophilia infections occurred nor for the year thereafter. What does the latter imply for the occurrence of seemingly sporadic S. maltophilia infections otherwise?

Figure 2. Fingerprint patterns of *S. maltophilia* isolates from an outbreak. Note homology of fingerprint patterns for three isolates.

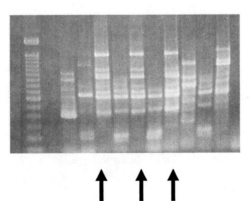

214

Figure 3. Schematic diagram of inter-repeat element PCR as a tool for molecular fingerprinting. See Chapter IV for a discussion of PCR (polymerase chain reaction). Bacterial DNA normally has a number of repeated sequences of DNA, often whose functions are not understood. These repeated sequences vary throughout the bacterial genome. Amplification of areas between these repeat sequences given variable length PCR products which, when resolved, give a fingerprint profile much like pulsed field gel electrophoresis (Figure 1) although the fragments are much smaller.

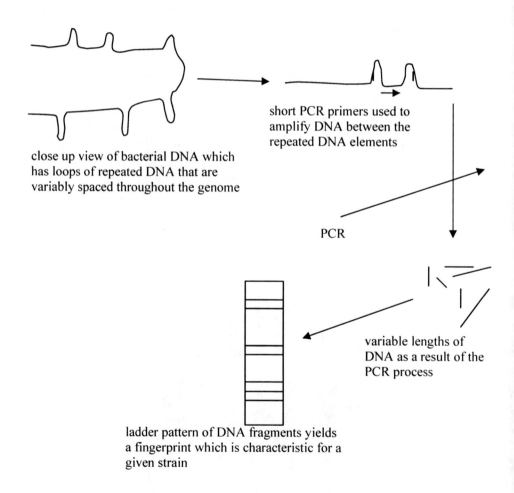

short PCR primers used to amplify DNA between the repeated DNA elements

close up view of bacterial DNA which has loops of repeated DNA that are variably spaced throughout the genome

PCR

variable lengths of DNA as a result of the PCR process

ladder pattern of DNA fragments yields a fingerprint which is characteristic for a given strain

From an infection control and public health perspective, fingerprinting has become an invaluble resource. It may not necessarily be required every day, but it has the power to support epidemiological investigations considerably. In the end, it still requires the astute observer and the inquiring mind to fit pieces of the puzzle together.

Food For Thought

1. Draw analogies between fingerprinting methods for human forensic purposes and for a bacterial outbreak. What differences might there be?
2. What is the difference between a bacterial 'strain', a bacterial 'isolate', a bacterial 'species', and a bacterial 'clone'?
3. When we generally think of outbreaks, we usually take it to mean that a single clone of germ is responsible for the disease. Could there be concurrent outbreaks of different germs in the same setting, either for the same or different types of infection? Could one encounter an outbreak setting with one species of germ (e.g., a bacterial species), but where there is more than one strain of the same germ?

Suggested Reading

Cimolai N, Trombley C, Wensley D, LeBlanc J. Heterogeneous *Serratia marcescens* genotypes from a nosocomial pediatric outbreak. *Chest* Vol. 111: pages 194-197 (1997).
- your answer to part of Question 3. above

Soll DR, Pujol C, Lockhart SR. Laboratory procedures for the epidemiological analysis of microorganisms. Chapter 11. *In*: Murray PR, Baron EJ, Jorgensen JH, Landry ML, Pfaller MA. *Manual of Clinical Microbiology*. 9th Edition. Washington, DC:ASM Press, 2007.
- exemplifies the diversity of current typing methods

Struelens M. Molecular epidemiology. Chapter 7. *In*: Cimolai N – ed. *Laboratory Diagnosis of Bacterial Infections*. New York, NY:Marcel Dekker, Inc., 2001.
- the science of how it is done

Tenover FC et al. How to select and interpret molecular typing methods for epidemiological studies of bacterial infections: a review for health care epidemiologists. *Infection Control and Hospital Epidemiology* Vol. 18: pages 426-439 (1997).
- a concise 'how to'

"The health of the people is really the foundation upon which all their happiness and all their powers as a state depend."
Benjamin Disraeli
Earl of Beaconsfield Speech, July 24, 1877

XVI. A Role for Public Health

What is Public Health?

'**Public health**' is a body of knowledge and participants of many that are dedicated to the protection and advancement of health among the general community. In achieving these goals, disease is understood, controlled, and prevented. By necessity, public health regards all aspects of health issues, and indeed it focuses on infectious diseases as a small but important subset. On a practical basis, however, much attention has been and continues to be focussed on infections. This arm of public health is perhaps best described as '**communicable disease control**'.

There is a necessary overlap between communicable disease control in the community and infection control programs of acute care settings. The former dwells on an interest in public health mainly with the common good for populations, whereas the latter is more likely to be applicable to mainly individuals in the setting of advanced diagnostics and therapeutics.

Even for communicable disease control, we can think of public health as a domain in a smaller community (e.g., town or city), but it is often referable to larger regions such as counties and provinces. Given the advances in travel, communicable diseases are highly mobile, and thus we must ultimately view public health in national and international terms.

Public Health Begins With Public Education

You cannot easily educate individuals or populations about infection control unless they have some fundamental and formal education. As such, public education for communicable diseases may be approached quite differently given the demographics and especially the level of education. It is extremely helpful to acute care settings when the individual patient or family member who is asked to participate in implementing an infection control technique has some rudimentary foundation in cleanliness and hygiene. For health care workers, the latter is generally assumed. In the setting of public health, it is evident that better education overall is associated with greater potential to manage and prevent infections. In turn, the standard of living for a given population is a major factor.

Education in personal and public hygiene should begin in the early ages and indeed become part of school curricula. It is hoped that such education is incremental and ultimately leads to a knowledgeable adult population whose behaviour is consistent with good communicable disease prevention. Among the many aspects of personal hygiene, handwashing is the most important, and it should accordingly be emphasized with even the most basic instructions.

Apart from the role of education in relationship to communicable disease prevention, it is becoming increasingly apparent that public health concerns with infection are more of an issue in the lay press. Reports of outbreaks, unusual infections, new discoveries, among other things have become very newsworthy items. The barrage of audio and visual media that we are exposed to ensures that such topics are encountered on a frequent basis. Some of this reporting is inadvertently misleading, often in respect to either the severity or magnitude of the problem. It is thus of benefit to have a population with a sense of preparedness and an expectation of the reality. Public health serves to educate co-participants in an active process rather than allow for reactionists who respond to everything.

A Mandate for Public Health

With the presence of infection control services in many acute care facilities, public health practitioners who report to regional authorities often have a limited role in this setting. Nevertheless, there are many benefits to having a good liaison between acute care and public health. Apart from informal interactions between the two parties, public health is often represented on acute care Infection Control Committees.

Outside of the acute setting, the mandate of public health becomes more obvious. There is no doubt that the form of health care system affects what degree of public health involvement there may be. In a comprehensive health care plan, providers may already have essential bridges between acute and chronic or community care as well as being able to respond to timely issues. In most populations, however, there is a need for public health authorities to assume full, or at least some ownership, for long-term care, home care, office care (including dentistry), and community outbreaks. Similar responsibility also spills over into schools and day care settings. Congregations of individuals in general, or furthermore those with particular risk factors, may especially serve as foci where certain communicable diseases are spread.

The provision of safe living conditions is a prerequisite to good personal and community hygiene. It is taken for granted by many that drinking water should be safe, and yet many outbreaks in well-developed countries continue to occur and even affect large populations. Food safety is also a major concern for public health, and food may serve as an important and common vehicle in modernized countries. For example, public health should have a role in monitoring communicable disease problems of food services (e.g., restaurants and other eateries) and food manufacturing (e.g., milk pasteurization). Table 1 details some specific examples of infection hazards in these areas.

Food-borne illnesses are particularly common in society, and they continue to be associated with much morbidity and mortality. Many of these can be prevented by adherence to simple and common food preparation and maintenance practices. Although perhaps obvious to many, the frequency at which food is prepared and the natural occurrence of error both contribute to a high probability that food-borne illnesses will occur.

Preventative health may require active treatment of infected individuals (e.g., a patient with diphtheria who is appropriately treated with an antibiotic will have reduced shedding of the pathogenic bacterium from the respiratory tract). Contacts of an active infection may also be suitable recipients of a prophylactic antibiotic therapy prior to the development of an infection so as to eliminate the carrier state or the pre-infection state (e.g., the direct family contacts of a patient with diphtheria will receive prophylaxis)(see Chapters IX and XIII). Prophylaxis in this context may take place in the way of a single individual, or it may involve numerous individuals especially in an outbreak (e.g., a small meningococcal outbreak in a school could conceivably warrant prophylaxis of the school cohort).

Table 1. Examples of human pathogens and illnesses that are associated with transmission in the context of poor living conditions, tainted water, and tainted food.

Poor living conditions	Tainted water	Tainted food
scabies	giardiasis	yersiniosis
lice	cryptosporidiosis	salmonellosis
Bartonella quintana	campylobacteriosis	*L. monocytogenes*
drug-use related infections	Legionnaire's Disease	trichinosis
leprosy	gastrointestinal viruses	botulism
tuberculosis	shigellosis	enterohemorrhagic
bed bugs	cholera	*E. coli*

The use of prophylactic agents has been guided by past experience and scientific trials, and it is applicable only to select infectious diseases.

Contact tracing is an important function for public health. In reference to antimicrobial prophylaxis as detailed above, further disease or chronic carriage as a reservoir can also be prevented. Indeed, some of the contacts may truly have silent infections (e.g., sexual contacts of a patient who has *Chlamydia trachomatis* genital infection may be actively ill or suffer unknowingly from an indolent asymptomatic infection); these contacts will be capable of spreading infection similar to the index case. As we have determined, antiviral prophylaxis is not of value in many circumstances, but yet the tracing of contacts may have other ramifications. On one hand, it may be of benefit to the patient to know of the exposure and its consequences for health reasons (e.g., the knowledge of tuberculosis contact may alert the individual and the health provider to future illness). On the other hand, the contact may lead to an actual infection (e.g., hepatitis B or C, HIV-infection, syphilis) which may not be initially recognized, but which is re-transmissible.

The administration of vaccines is variably conducted by private practitioners and public health clinics or employees. The latter is influenced by the particular organization of the health care system. Regardless of specific provider, the organization of vaccine programs and recommendations often rests with the public health authorities. The existing and emerging vaccines have provided a wealth of work in this area (see Chapter XIII).

Often by legislation, public health authorities are commanded to tabulate the occurences of various infectious diseases. The latter are often termed 'reportable diseases', and the reporting is initiated by primary practitioners and/or laboratories. Whereas most reportable diseases have a laboratory diagnostic method as their basis, some may be reportable on the basis of a clinical syndrome only (e.g., pertussis). The inclusions among reportable diseases are variable depending on the geographic locale, but many preventable and infectious illnesses are often standard among such lists (e.g., tuberculosis, gonorrhea, botulism). Table 2 outlines some commonly reportable diseases. In part, such reporting facilitates the understanding of trends in communicable diseases. Thus, the surveillance system must be consistent in ascertaining and reporting. Many reportable diseases are indeed preventable, and thus problems with prevention strategies may be seen as well when they fail.

Standards of quarantine for infections in the public domain are also generally under the purview of public health. At times, it is apparent that some standards which are otherwise stringently enforced in an acute care setting must be appropriately modified in consideration of the realities of the community. As

Table 2. Reportable communicable diseases (note: these may vary from region to region).

AIDS	Anthrax	Botulism
Brucellosis	Chancroid	*C. trachomatis*
Cholera	*Cryptosporidium*	Diphtheria
Encephalitis and meningitis	Selected enteric bacterial	Giardia
Gonorrhea	pathogens (e.g. *Campylobacter,*	Invasive *S. pyogenes*
Invasive *Haemophilus influenzae*	*Salmonella, Shigella, Yersinia*	Hantavirus
Hemolytic-Uremic Syndrome	*enterocolitica,* enterohemorrhagic	Leprosy
Measles	*E. coli*)	Invasive meningococci
Mumps	Pertussis	Plague
Polio	Rabies	Rubella
SARS	Syphilis	Tetanus
Toxic shock syndrome	Trichinosis	Tuberculosis
Typhoid fever		

in acute care settings, the public health authorities must exercise risk management.

If not only by reviewing the list of reportable communicable diseases, it is apparent that the mandate of public health is quite broad in regards to infection. On a practical basis, however, there are common problems which predominate. Among several, these include food poisoning, head lice, sexually transmitted diseases and AIDS, influenza, tuberculosis, meningococcal infection, and infections of travel. The topic of antibiotic resistant bacteria is becoming increasingly important especially as these problems spread to the community from acute care settings. The latter issue may very well force public health to intervene, if not only seriously examine antibiotics in general.

Standards for employee health and in general occupational health and safety are often influenced, if not managed, by public health. Public health often has a role regarding vector-borne diseases (e.g., insect transmitted) and their control via public health measures (e.g., insecticide use). The incidence of environmental infections (e.g., Legionnaire's disease) can be affected by public health measures (e.g., recommendations for potable water storage or construction of buildings). Monitoring of zoonoses and geographic diseases may also be relevant.

Biological terrorism is a new concept to many, and the thoughts of its potential have been ever so apparent in the lay press. Although the concept is certainly not new, the use of biological weapons as an adjunct to more physical components of warfare has raised the anxiety of all nations. Potential biological weapons include the dissemination to populations of anthrax, plague, Q fever, brucellosis, smallpox, and botulism toxin. Perhaps most concerning amongst this potential is the ever increasing spread of knowledge and thus capability among members of the world communities. In this regard, public health authorities have recently enhanced surveillance systems and have redefined mechanisms for an effective response. Public education is equally important.

As public health authorities often have equally important reporting to regional and larger governments, there is the potential to significantly influence public health care spending. For the benefit of acute care settings or others, the public health mandate can be an essential ally.

Food For Thought

1. Postulate the components and mechanisms of delivery for a public health campaign which is aimed at the prevention of food-borne infections among the community at large.
2. Examine the methods which are used to provide potable water to the public. Where in these systems do germs enter?
3. Table 1 outlines a few examples of infections that may be a function of poor living conditions. What other infections may be associated with poor socioeconomic status?
4. What infections are considered quarantineable in the community?

Suggested Reading

Detels R, et al. – eds. *Oxford Textbook of Public Health.* 5th Edition. New York, NY:Oxford University Press, 2009.
- a multi-volume encyclopedic treasury

McKenzie JF, Pinger RR, Kotecki JE. *An Introduction to Community Health.* 7th Edition. Boston, MA:Jones and Bartlett, 2011.
- a comprehensive introduction

Noji EK. *The Public Health Consequences of Disasters.* New York, NY:Oxford University Press, 1997.
- infection has a major role

Parker R, Sommer M - eds. *Routledge Handbook in Global Public Health.* Oxon, UK:Routledge, 2011.
- taking a broader glance in the global context

Rutherford GW. Public health, communicable diseases, and managed care: will managed care improve or weaken communicable disease control? *American Journal of Preventive Medicine* Vol. 14 (Supplement 3): pages 53-59 (1998).
- read this in retrospect and determine whether the author's theses were well predicated

" ... growth of the mind is the widening
of the range of consciousness, and that each
step forward has been a most painful and
laborious achievement."
> Carl Gustav Jung
> *Contributions to Analytical Psychology*, 1928

XVII. Plagues of Our Times

Old Diseases, New Diseases, Increasing Interests

Ancient writings from all corners of the world document epidemics of infection that have affected large populations and have dramatically changed the history of the world. Perhaps most of these will never have an etiological agent clearly defined, but certainly the scourges of smallpox, plague, influenza, and tuberculosis come to obvious attention. The cyclical nature of illnesses was also evident, and in the pre-antibiotic era, there were few interventions that had much impact. Antibiotics and vaccination dramatically changed the pattern of many infectious diseases over the last five decades especially to the point where indeed some of these are rarities in modernized countries (e.g., diphtheria, tetanus).

Despite contemporary times and associated progress, epidemics continue. Many of these are due to pathogens which continue to cause sporadic disease in the same populations. Even for infectious diseases which are in declining frequency, a pattern of decline may yet be superimposed by periodic outbreaks as long as the pathogen and vehicle(s) for transmission remain. The latter is analogous to the changing fortunes of a stock market which is subject to increases and decreases although the overall trend may average upward or downward over a given longer period of time.

Naturally, our expectations initially, and into the future, are that infectious diseases should decline, but there are several reasons why this area continues to weigh heavily in the minds of physicians and scientists. Firstly, there has been tremendous progress over the last three decades, and new etiological agents have been defined (e.g., HIV, Lyme disease, hepatitis C, and *Ehrlichia* spp., etc.)(see Table 1) Whereas these agents and their infections have likely been affecting the human race for a long time, their novelty has subsequently led to an explosion of information which would make it seem that such infections are truly new. Secondly, some previously recognized infections have re-emerged in their

224

Table 1. New etiological agents of infection from the 1990s illustrating how quickly new understandings emerge.

1999- West Nile virus, New York state
    Influenza A H9N2, Hong Kong
1998- Nipah virus
1997- enterovirus 71
    transfusion-transmitted virus (TTV)
    Influenza A H5N1, Hong Kong
1996- prion, new variant CJD
1995- Hendra virus

1994- human herpesvirus 8
    Sabia virus, Brazil
1993- hepatitis G
    Sin nombre virus (new Hantavirus)
1992- *Bartonella henselae*
1991- hepatitis F
1990- hepatitis E
    human herpesvirus 7

Table 2. Emerging infectious diseases of the last three decades.

Cholera
Clostridium difficile diarrhea
Cryptosporidium
Dengue fever
Drug-resistant staphylococci, enterococci, coliform gram negative rods
Drug-resistant tuberculosis
Enterohemorrhagic *E. coli* (e.g. *E. coli* O157:H7)
Hantavirus
Helicobacter pylori
Hepatitis C
Human immunodeficiency virus (HIV)
Influenza (new variants)

Legionnaire's disease
Lyme disease
Malaria
Norwalk-like agents
Pertussis
Prions - spongiform encephalopathy [(BSE) of cattle; Creutzfeldt-Jakob disease (CJD) of humans]
Salmonella
SARS-CoV
Schistosomiasis
Staphylococcal toxic shock
Viral hemorrhagic fevers (Lassa, Ebola, Argentinian, Bolivian)
Yellow fever

prominence. Whether this has occurred as a natural cyclical phenomenon or whether there have been specific precipitants in recent times remain the subject for investigation in each case. Thirdly, for some endemic infections, the frequencies may not so much have changed, but rather some phenotypic trait may have emerged that creates additional concern above and beyond the usual. The latter might include changes of increased virulence or antibiotic resistance. Overall, we now often refer to this net incremental change as '**emerging**

infectious diseases'. These infections have thus either newly appeared or have existed but are seemingly and rapidly increasing in incidence or geographic spread. Table 2 gives examples of these plagues of our times. Among these emerging infections, several have a direct link to hospital settings and are greatly influenced by the power of infection control programs (e.g., MRSA, *C. difficile*, vancomycin-resistant enterococci, drug-resistant tuberculosis).

What can account for emerging infectious diseases? Outside of these pathogens which are indeed newly discovered and therefore novel only on this basis, it is evident at times that precipitating factors especially include those which are of demographic, environmental, or ecological nature, and which enhance the probability of interaction between microbe and host or simply promote transmission. Natural or selected changes in microbial genomes also allow the microbe to change in appearance or virulence.

Changes in the environment, or the way we interact with the environment, have altered the pattern of interactions between pathogen and host. For example, global climatic changes were touted to have increased water temperatures and to favour epidemic cholera in the Americas. Agricultural and water ecosystem changes have favoured infections like schistosomiasis.

There have been many events in the demographics and behaviour of societies, large or small, that have fostered some infections and their spread. For example, population shifts of emigration and war have led to an admixture of susceptible and non-susceptible. Urbanization, changes in sexual mores, and intravenous drug use all have their associations with specific infections.

Globalization and industry too have their problems. Food is now disseminated globally in short order and in a pattern that exposes large populations. Advancing medical practice brings with it the hazards of new approaches and technologies. Antibiotics have increasingly been used for humans but as well for the animal industries. Human-sourced medical products created major problems with world-wide spread of hepatitis C and HIV.

A negative change in public health provisions given particular circumstances has also been a major factor. The former Soviet Union, for example, suffered from outbreaks of diphtheria as vaccination programs were lacking during a period of economic and social upheaval. The rapid development of refugee camps in many parts of the world is associated with poor hygienic measures, inadequate health care, and crowding. Inadequately treated tuberculosis favoured the emergence of drug resistance.

We cannot underestimate the role of travel in the dissemination of infection. Whereas the majority of such travel is due to international travelers who are mobile for family, pleasure, and work, immigration and refugee migration are also important aspects. From the perspective of travel medicine, returning travelers, who have spent considerable periods of time with family members in underdeveloped regions of the world, are not uncommonly in need of medical care. Airplanes themselves offer a small opportunity for the mobilization of insect vectors, but more commonly, travellers have already acquired the infection in the country of visit, and immigrants and refugees are already infected when they cross borders. Malaria, dengue fever, and yellow fever represent some of the more common infections of travel. Infectious gastroenteritis is experienced by a large number of travellers depending on the destination, and this underscores the importance of safe food and water.

Microbial evolution cannot be underestimated. The inherent ability to change through mutation and selection of the fittest allows for adaptation, and thereafter allows for an emergence potentially of enhanced virulence. The environment, the body and its immunity, and antimicrobials all influence the selective process. Ongoing but minor and sudden dramatic changes in influenza viruses and the outbreak potential of such consequences reflect a prime example of this theme. One only needs to look at the significant pandemic with H1N1 of the last few years. For decades, it was suggested that natural selection would promote a trade-off with the outcome of a benign equilibrium between the microbe and the human. We now realize that such an equilibrium will be destabilized when the microbe exploits the human through success over cycles of transmission and with a greater success than a microbe will have in any form of mutual co-existence. Ultimately, the evolution of virulence will be a trade-off between the competitive phases accommodated through disease versus any harmful effect to transmission that occurs when the outcome of infection reduces contact between the ill patient and the next susceptible one.

A Framework for Control

Given the above concerns and the implications for contagion to spread beyond the boundaries of localized regions, national and international policies must be developed so that effective monitoring is established and so that emergency response plans can be activated in a co-ordinated and timely fashion.

On an international scale, the World Health Organization (WHO) establishes a legal and policy framework for addressing the issue of epidemic global spread. International agreements on trade and sanitary measures have some impact in having the WHO actions enforced. Nevertheless, such regulations are in need of revision due to the ever-changing priorities in emerging infections, and a more cohesive method to combat emerging infections globally is still needed. These efforts must overcome problems of economic change and turmoil, civil unrest, monetary debt, natural global phenomena such as disasters and weather change, and simple complacency especially of those countries that have resources to make a difference.

Communications and People

From the perspective of medical authorities and public health support, the organization of response plans is perhaps the more straightforward. Communication to the public is another matter however and indeed a source of much confusion. This confusion is fueled by a variable level of education and hence understanding, incomplete information, second-hand knowledge, and at times, fear. Effective communication theory must be activated in order for the public to appreciate the issue, perhaps participate in active control, and certainly to avoid creating more problems whether imagined or real.

The source of information to be delivered must be balanced and accurate. The message must be carefully constructed, and the target audience(s) should be realized. Often, a combination of strategies must be undertaken.

Communications for the masses must often be channeled through the common media. Accordingly, the media themselves must be educated. It is of very little value to have a clear statement forwarded which will be unfortunately misstated and twisted by those who may be expert in communication but short on medical science. Information on this large scale can be organized through various mass media campaigns, news media, and even popular entertainment modes.

Future Shock

In many ways, the future is unpredictable, but we are not globally powerless in the fight against infection. We must expand our knowledge of those factors that lead to disease emergence. The establishment of global surveillance is a necessary first step. We may initially focus on the containment of more virulent microbes rather than on the suppression of any given emerging disease. Nevertheless, even in this light, we must attempt to curtail both microbes that are clearly recognized as obvious threats, and as well, those that are yet to be fully recognized.

Plagues of Our Times

As we have previously discussed, there are many emerging infections that have captivated the attention of the medical community. By example, we illustrate aspects of infection emergence using the specific citations of MRSA, hepatitis C, Lyme disease, and SARS.

MRSA

Staphylococcus aureus has long been recognized as a very important human pathogen and for some a commensal in the upper respiratory tract and occasionally skin. It was not until the 1930s that much could be done to fight infections when sulphonamides became available as the first major group of antibiotics. By the early 1940s, penicillin G became available, and it was very much a boon to medicine initially, but by the end of the same decade, resistance to penicillin G became problematic as increasing numbers of isolates possessed an ability to produce penicillinase or beta-lactamase (a degrading enzyme). Subsequently, newer staphylococcal agents became available such as tetracyclines, erythromycin, and streptomycin, but the use of the latter too was associated with quickly emerging resistance.

It was desirable to develop beta-lactam antibiotics (see Chapter IX) for several reasons, and indeed two variations of such antibiotics which were resistant to the staphylococcal beta-lactamase became available. The first group of these included the antibiotics methicillin, oxacillin, and dicloxacillin. Within a few years, the second group that emerged was the cephalosporins ('first generation', e.g., cefazolin; see Chapter IX). The beta-lactam antibiotics were extremely important innovations, and in many contexts they continue to remain highly effective and pragmatic choices. Nevertheless, 'methicillin resistance' became evident within a year after clinical use of the first group in the United Kingdom. Although termed 'methicillin resistance' because methicillin was being used clinically and because its susceptibility was tested for, resistance was found to all agents of the latter antibiotic groups. The term 'MRSA' has remained with us as a consequence of the latter even though methicillin itself is not commonly used.

Initially, the occurrence of MRSA seemed sporadic, but eventually outbreaks were experienced. These were often contained, and alternate antibiotics were still efficacious. Two critical trends appeared within the decade of the 1960s. Firstly, some MRSA isolates acquired other antibiotic resistances. Although at first only one or two other resistances were observed, eventually strains emerged which bore resistance to many more other available antibiotics with few exceptions. The latter multi-resistant bacteria were given the lay designation '**superbugs**'. The second important trend was the occurrence if not dissemination on a world-wide basis. Outside of the United Kingdom, major problems with MRSA were evident in Australia and the United States. In the United States for example, MRSA was first reported in the early 1960s. To this day, there are few countries that have been relatively spared, and major regional outbreaks continue to be reported. Although countries may have considerable variation between region, morbidity and mortality due to MRSA are commonplace. Linkages have been determined among some strains that are found in different regions, indeed continents. In the last decade alone, a pandemic of highly virulent MRSA, that is commonly associated with community-acquired soft tissue infrections, has emerged.

Although MRSA often do possess the penicillinase enzyme, their resistance to other beta-lactam antibiotics occurs as a consequence of another mechanism. When penicillin-like antibiotics interact with a bacterium, they are active at a site where the bacterial cell wall is forming. Here they bind to structures, mainly proteins, that facilitate cell wall synthesis, and thus, a susceptible bacterium will in essence self-destruct as the rigid cell wall boundary is unable to form. For MRSA, the component at the site of cell wall synthesis that normally binds cloxacillin, for example, is altered; the alteration diminishes the ability of the antibiotic to achieve the aforementioned effect. The nature of this resistance changes the way almost all beta-lactam antibiotics bind to the bacterium, and thus they are all somewhat compromised in their ability to neutralize the pathogen. The occurrence of resistance to other antibiotics is variable and is acquired. Among MRSA in areas where the resistance has newly occurred (i.e., the bacterium is not imported from another setting), there may only be methicillin resistance. As MRSA are exposed repetitively to other agents, resistance becomes cumulative. The mechanisms for all of these resistances can be quite different and do not occur as a consequence of the changes that are evident at the site of penicillin binding. MRSA that are resistant to almost all other options, except for vancomycin and some topical antibiotics, have become real acute care concerns.

When one compares MRSA isolates in general with fully antibiotic susceptible *S. aureus*, it has been generally believed that a difference in virulence is not evident. Whereas this may be correct with respect to the generalities between two large populations of bacteria, it may not necessarily be true for a given strain. Even among antibiotic susceptible *S. aureus* isolates, it has been known for decades that some strains are more pathogenic than others. Likewise, it is possible that a given MRSA strain is more virulent than other MRSA isolates, and thus, it is also credible that some MRSA may be more virulent than some or many antibiotic susceptible *S. aureus*. MRSA that are endemic to hospitals and that have been circulating among and infecting patients may indeed have greater virulence through a selection process. The control of MRSA in some circumstances may thus be indicated due to the impact on treatment options but as well due to the potential for more disease after colonization.

From an outside perspective, one may view susceptibility testing as a laboratory procedure that should be relatively simple and that should be available and reproducible even decades ago. Unfortunately, this has not been the case. Many centres world-wide did not even test *S. aureus* for 'methicillin' resistance. When methods for doing so were developing, there was considerable variation in their application. Although susceptibility testing methods are generally manual, automated methods for susceptibility testing became popular, but they were fraught with difficulty especially with an inability to detect resistance when it was present. Conditions for reliably detecting such resistance indeed proved to be significant variations from those methods that are otherwise used to routinely test *S. aureus* for susceptibility to other antibiotics. Furthermore, it proved that *S. aureus* isolates could be heterogeneously resistant (i.e., not all bacteria in a laboratory culture express their resistance fully), and this phenomenon proved to be a barrier to the definition of a reliable methodology. Although MRSA detection is more consistent in the current era among laboratories, it is reasonable to believe that historic problems in this regard may have contributed to spread since some MRSA were simply not being recognized. The latter illustrates how critical it is to have precision technologies.

As previously emphasized, MRSA colonization rates among patients in acute care and chronic care facilities have generally increased, and some institutions have staggering frequencies of MRSA (among all hospital *S. aureus* isolates) approaching 50% or more. An accompaniment of such increase has been a proportionate rise in the frequency of nosocomial MRSA infections. The complications of the latter have been considerably varied. Whereas most MRSA acquisitions are but mere colonizations of the skin and/or upper respiratory tract, advanced morbidity (e.g., septic shock, central nervous system infection) and indeed mortality are real concerns and now not uncommon for some institutions. Risk factors for acquisition of MRSA vary depending on the setting, but include long term care, chronic antibiotic use, exposure to other known MRSA-positive patients or MRSA-endemic institutions, presence of foreign materials (e.g., gastric tube, intravenous devices), chronic wounds or skin conditions, poor functional status of the patient, adult intensive and transplantation care, among other things.

Is control of MRSA at the institutional level worth it? Of course it is, but we must view current controversies in this regard with some perspective. For facilities that are clear or relatively spared, a comparatively small effort and minimal resources may be required. The costs of endemic MRSA in acute care may be impressive. In chronic care settings, much less impact of actual MRSA infection is felt, and therefore, much less interest is generated even when colonization rates are high. What is less understood, however, is that the chronic care facility may simply act as a reservoir for MRSA to be introduced back to acute care facilities. The nature of chronic care requires that many patient procedures be performed elsewhere, and patients in chronic care already have a higher risk for acute care needs. These return and re-entry events between facilities provide ample opportunity for MRSA spread from carriers. What may amount to a nuisance for a chronic care setting may well prove to be a disaster-in-waiting for the recipient of acute care. Furthermore, it is of some help when patients are known to be MRSA carriers, but such knowledge may not be known for a chronic care contact who has unknowingly acquired MRSA from an index case. For an acute care institution that has major problems with endemic MRSA, it may reach a point where desirable isolation precautions are untenable with such a large group. The physical layout and resources are important, but staff inertia and complacency may complicate matters more when problems are persistent. Health care professionals would rather see the entire problem solved rather than a temporary or permanent reduction, and they may be frustrated when even the best of efforts leads to some modest but not total improvement. Some facilities that continue to suffer from the wrath of MRSA, and who may have formerly been quite stringent about MRSA, now may opt for a two-tiered approach: a certain threshold of MRSA may be tolerated especially in areas of lesser acuity where infection control precautions are minimal, but more advanced precautions may be instituted and highly enforced in high risk areas where the consequences of colonization and infection are profound. There is convincing evidence that efforts to control MRSA will in most circumstances be associated with cost savings. How do we appropriately measure suffering and death? In any event, MRSA control is worth it, but the circumstances will dictate how control may be promoted and achieved. Little is it recognized that health care settings with MRSA problems are accountable for a spill-over effect into the general community. Community-acquired MRSA infections are now a reality and increasingly common in most areas. Some high risk groups (e.g., intravenous drug users) may be prone to such infections. These too will now serve as a reservoir for spread in the health care setting.

How do we control MRSA? Given the above discussion, we cannot view control as the mission of acute care settings only. The intensity of efforts may be greater in acute care, but the continuum of care necessitates a role for acute care, chronic care, home care, ambulatory care, and public health. For patients who are known to carry MRSA, appropriate precautions and quarantine are a must. Care in a single bed room is important. At a minimum, contact or barrier precautions should be implemented; some may use strict isolation given the potential for some airborne spread, although the latter is less common. A surveillance for MRSA is of value. Microbiological support should include appropriate methods for detection and susceptibility testing. Screening of admissions for carriage may be useful if patients come from high risk areas or other institutions. Follow-up and delisting criteria are of value for MRSA-positive patients who continue to require care after discharge. Acknowledgement of spread potentially via inanimate objects is critical. All too often, it is believed that spread can only occur by direct contact with a colonized patient. Environmental services are a key therefore to success in many aspects. Whereas patients may be carriers, less often health care workers may be the vehicle for transmission; a consideration for their detection and perhaps decolonization is important. Treatment of active MRSA infections often includes the use of vancomycin alone or in combination with other agents, and the outcome is usually a good one. Unfortunately, such systemic therapy does not commonly terminate colonization so that the potential for transmission can remain both during and after therapy. Progress in the control of antimicrobial use, and furthermore its reduction, are imperative.

Hepatitis C

Apart from the recognized infectious causes of hepatitis (commonly hepatitis A and B), it was noted decades ago that some apparently blood-transmitted hepatitides were likely being caused by an unrecognized agent. The disease entity was initially called **non-A, non-B hepatitis,** and an infectious agent theory was advanced and supported by numerous data. It was not until the latter part of the 1980s, however, that advanced molecular investigations proved the agent to be a novel virus, thereafter termed hepatitis C virus. This finding was certainly a magnificent discovery in large part due to the manner in which it was made. Laboratory animals had been infected by infusions of human factor VIII concentrate (clotting factor for hemophiliac use) which presumably contained the non-A, non-B agent. Without actually having isolated the whole virus from these animals, a portion of the genetic material (RNA) from this virus was 'cloned' from their blood. Products of these cloning experiments then became available for use in diagnostic methods of antibody detection. Thus, the infection was being indirectly detected even before it could be isolated in the laboratory, and even to this day, routine viral culture procedures do not permit whole virus detection. The availability of a diagnostic assay allowed for the elaboration of the epidemiology in a very short time. It now appears that hepatitis C is and was the most common cause of non-A, non-B hepatitis (there are a few others), is the infectious cause of most unexplained advanced liver failures (cirrhosis), is associated with liver cancer, and is the most common cause of liver failures that leads to liver transplantation.

The virus is much unlike other hepatitis viruses. In addition, there are several distinct subtypes of the virus; some of these may have somewhat different behaviour among patients. This variability also has the potential to allow evasion of host immune responses, and particular subtypes may be less responsive to antiviral therapy. Diagnostic tests must incorporate ways to detect these variations. Vaccine development may in part be hampered by such diversity.

Initial diagnostic tests were fraught with some difficulty in interpretation, but current methods have overcome much of these problems. Within a very short period of time, however, and despite any such difficulties, the epidemiology of infection became quickly understood. Frequencies of positive hepatitis C serology among blood donors have been approximately 0.5% in western countries, and the frequency approaches 0.5-2% in the general population. In some regions of Africa, however, the endemic rate of positive serology may be as high as 5%. Patients on renal dialysis have historically had rates of up to 20%, and frequencies are very high among sexual partners of infected patients and then also among intravenous drug abusers. The transmission of hepatitis C is somewhat analogous to hepatitis B. Contact with blood and body fluids confers most risk, and thus risk factors include: intravenous drug use, recipient of blood products, hemodialysis, organ transplant, needlestick injuries, high risk sexual activity, and being subject to body piercing or tattoos. Transmission from mother to infant does occur. With the use of molecular detection techniques, viral genome has been found in blood, body fluids, semen, saliva, and urine. Transmission by direct contact with an infected individual does not appear to present a risk unless there is a mechanism for more direct contact with blood and body fluids which have higher viral content.

After contact with the virus, an incubation period may vary from two weeks to five months (usually six to seven weeks). Most infections are seemingly asymptomatic, and clinical illness is usually mild when it occurs; a minority of patients actually develop an acute hepatitis which leads to jaundice. Only rarely does advanced and fulminant liver disease occur early in the illness. Therefore, among most infected patients, the illness may be determined early only when there are biochemical markers from blood tests which are performed to measure liver cell injury. Although antibodies to the virus do develop after the initial infection, these do not seem to be protective, and therefore these seem only useful to indicate that an infection has occurred. Most patients who become infected will stay infected for a life-time. In the absence of acute illnesses, patients are nevertheless still at risk for morbidity from ongoing complications. A chronic hepatitis can cause ongoing liver damage, and marked scarring and destruction of the liver may result in cirrhosis; the time for such complications is usually measured in many years (e.g., 20-25). Chronic scarring and other underlying changes in the liver may lead to liver cancer (hepatocellular carcinoma). Diseases of kidney, skin, and blood may also accompany chronic hepatitis C infection. Liver disease may be compounded by a concomitant infection with hepatitis B. Advanced liver failure may require liver transplantation, if it is available. Overall, the mechanisms of virus persistence, replication, and ongoing liver injury are not very well understood. It is evident from the numbers presented herein that hepatitis C causes considerable morbidity world-wide.

The first generation of diagnostic tools was designed to detect antibody as a marker of infection. These were designed with the principles of screening and confirmatory tests (see Chapter IV; Serology). On occasion, these tests may be indeterminate, but positive serology correlates very well with active infection. In addition, new molecular techniques have become available to measure virus RNA, and these may be applied to blood samples to confirm the diagnosis and to quantitate changes in the viral load if an antiviral therapy is contemplated.

Several antiviral agents have been found to affect hepatitis C replication, and these have been used alone or in combination to attempt treatment. A favourable response occurs for some individuals, and many of these will relapse after the course of therapy is finished. Therapy is also not uncommonly accompanied by side effects. The treatment studies are promising, and indeed treatment does seemingly cure a modest number of patients. Nevertheless, there is much to be learned here, and the issues of what agents to use, for how long to treat, and for which likely patients will benefit remain to be fully clarified. A good starting point has been initiated.

The lack of a good prevention strategy during times of exposure is disappointing. At least in the case of hepatitis B, vaccination as well as hepatitis B immune globulin are of significant benefit. Essentially then, prevention is a function of general recommendations to prevent exposure and universal screening programs for blood donors.

Lyme disease

'Lyme disease' is caused by several species of spirochetal (twisting spiral morphology) bacteria that belong to the genus *Borrelia*, and the best known of these is *Borrelia burgdorferi*. Illnesses caused by *Borrelia* species are generically called borrelioses. Prior to the recognition of Lyme disease, another borreliosis had been recognized for decades before. It is termed 'relapsing fever', and it is a recurrent febrile illness with few other manifestations and is associated with the presence of blood-borne spirochetes during these febrile episodes. Lyme disease, however, can be an illness which includes several body organs. Lyme disease was more fully understood in the 1980s after the major etiological agent, *B. burgdorferi*, was discovered in the United States. The history of Lyme disease appears to be a very contemporary one given that the latter finding occurred only some three decades ago. In North America, the discovery mainly began with a recognition that an arthritis among children not uncommonly was associated with a tick bite in a local area of Connecticut state. Some of those children also suffered with a particular skin rash especially at the site of tick bite. Culture of affected tissue yielded a new bacterium which resembled previously known spirochetes called *Borrelia* species. Thereafter, the availability of the bacterium in the laboratory allowed for the development of diagnostic tests which facilitated an understanding of disease spectrum and epidemiology.

At first, it appeared that the infections were essentially confined to endemic areas of northwest United States, but endemic areas were soon found throughout the United States, and equivalently endemic areas began to be apparent throughout Europe and other continents. In retrospect, it is known that the clinical illnesses of Lyme disease had been described in Sweden and France many decades back. It is now evident that hundreds of thousands of such infections have been reported world-wide.

Lyme disease is a zoonosis, and the pathogenic bacteria are transmitted to human by hard ticks mainly represented by the group known as *Ixodes* species. The specific *Ixodes* species of tick that is responsible for spread varies among geographic locales. Although the main bacterium causing Lyme disease was coined as *B. burgdorferi*, we now recognize that various other species may cause the same disease world-wide. For example, in Europe, there are currently three main species involved in disease: *B. burgdorferi*, *B. afzelii*, and *B. garinii*. These spirochetal bacteria infect mammals in nature, but the transfer of infection remains the function of ticks. The bacteria multiply in ticks, and the ticks may carry them through their life cycle. Furthermore, the bacteria may be transferred from the adult tick to its eggs for the next generation. Ticks search for a blood feed from mammals, and in nature, the subjects may be small mammals such as rodents or large animals such as deer (Figure 1). Young nymphal ticks are more likely to infect the small mammals since the small ticks are less mobile, whereas adult and more mobile ticks creep onto vegetation and latch on to larger mammals. When ticks burrow through mammalian skin, they draw a blood feed, but they may simultaneously regurgitate inner contents which contain the bacterium, and thus infection may be initiated. Geographic regions vary in the density of ticks that may be found; this density often correlates with the risk of acquiring Lyme disease. Furthermore, the frequency of tick infestation by Lyme spirochetes is also quite variable but usually includes only a minority of the ticks. Given the life cycle of ticks in nature, winter seasons in temperate climates are

Figure 1. Life cycle of ticks.

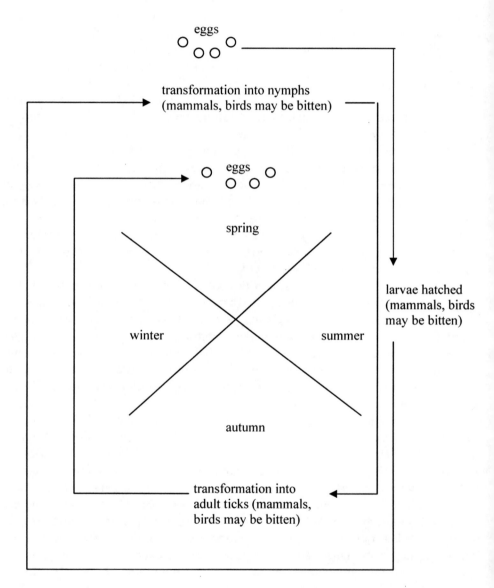

usually free of transmission, and transmission is more likely to occur during spring and summer seasons when tick activity, and likely interaction with tick infested environments, is greatest. Birds too may carry ticks and spirochetes. Whereas it is conceivable that mammalian infection with Lyme disease spirochetes existed for centuries past, it is realistic that human migration, with its associated land development and urbanization, have also increased the potential for such contact.

Lyme disease spirochetes are quite unique among bacteria. They are very difficult to culture in the laboratory, and they are not found by routine culture methods. Hence, diagnosis is most often accomplished by detecting antibody responses. These bacteria are also unique in that they are capable of changing their outer most membrane, or coat, during the course of an infection. Thus, while the immune response may initially recognize the outside of the bacterium and raise an attack against the bacterium, the bacteria change their appearance and thereafter evade any such immune response. This variability in bacterial appearance thus allows the infection to persist for long periods.

Lyme disease is noted for its involvement of skin, joints, nervous system, and heart. The progression of illness occurs in stages from superficial to disseminated and possibly chronic infection. At the site of tick bite, there may be very little reaction at all. Many infiltrations by Lyme spirochetes will be handled by the body, and no infection will occur thereafter. For others, the local inoculation will be followed by a local skin rash called 'erythema chronicum migrans'. This rash is a centrifugally expanding red rash, and most commonly is apparent within 1-2 weeks of the tick bite. Most patients will not recall a tick bite probably due to the small size of the tick. Although the infection may be limited to the tick bite focus, local or blood-borne spread may occur, and thus other body sites become infected. Neurological illness is quite variable, but it can involve peripheral nerves, the lining of the central nervous system, or the central nervous system itself. Joint and muscle aches may occur as well as actual arthritis; according to some, a few patients may experience a chronic arthritis. Involvement of the heart can lead to irregular heart beats and contractions. Differences in the degree of body involvement may also occur with the different species of *Borrelia* as well as with different strains of the same species. Fortunately, antibiotic therapy is of value for many forms of these illnesses.

Early in our understanding of Lyme disease, accurate diagnosis was a problem, and indeed it was believed that considerable over-diagnosis was occurring. Diagnostic tests have improved considerably, and much more accuracy is now possible. Blood tests are screened for an antibody response which, if positive, is confirmed by more advanced approaches.

238

Vaccines are now in some limited use but do not appear to have, as yet, a major role in prevention. Avoidance of ticks in endemic areas is perhaps most important. Person-to-person transmission does not occur, and this infection is certainly not a nosocomial hazard.

Lyme disease is therefore a zoonosis which exemplifies the issue of emergence, having newly recognized the causative agent only three decades ago, and now having a wealth of knowledge regarding the bacterium, epidemiology, disease associations, diagnosis, and treatment.

SARS

Coronaviruses were recognized as early as the 1930s, although of relevance seemingly then only to veterinary disease. By the early 1960s, however, human derived strains were determined to be causes of respiratory infection akin to the common cold. Research in this field was hampered by the inability of the diagnostic laboratory to easily recognize these viruses in clinical specimens.

In November, 2002, a cluster of viral-like respiratory illnesses emerged among individuals in the Guangdong province of China. The illness was quickly spread eastern Asia-wide and then globally. The disease was largely characterized by an influenza-like illness which typically included fever, malaise, rigors, and fatigue. In some, there was rapid progression to pneumonia and/or other severe pulmonary afflictions. Both the morbidity and mortality were high among those infected. Of note, the infection was less aggressive in young children, but it carried considerable morbidity for those older than 60 years.

By February, 2003, a causative agent had been identified as a new variant of coronaviruses. The latter finding was critical towards the development of relevant diagnostic methods for virus detection, but equally important was the epidemiological finding that many early infections in China had occurred among animal handlers, especially those frequenting large markets where animals were sold. Further investigation established a strong linkage with 'masked palm civets' (a furry small mammal) which had been sold in these markets for food. The civets proved only to be intermediates, much like humans, and the natural source of the virus has proven likely to be Chinese horseshoe bats. Effectively, the outbreak occurred as a consequence of animal to human transmission given the circumstances which prevailed in China.

The outbreak worldwide ended by 2004, although another small resurgence of infection occurred in China when wild animal trading resumed in such marketplaces. The virus is believed to have been spread via aerosol and through fecal-oral transmission. There were very high rates of secondary transmission among healthcare workers, even when infection control precautions were maintained. The virus was found to survive in fomites and stool for up to 24-72 hours. Aerosol transmission was highly suspect in some clusters of infection, and thus efficient fitted personal protective equipment was touted. Many sought to restrict patients to negative pressure ventilated rooms and under strict precautions (see Chapter VII). Some have suggested that the outbreak may have stopped since human infection may be an end-stage for the virus, and it was not clear that infection control interventions were clearly responsible for containment.

Intense research that accompanied this outbreak led to the discovery of other new human coronaviruses that have seemingly less virulence. It is remarkable how an animal source virus could lead to such rapid human spread and morbidity. Indeed, the global reaction to the appearance and recognition of SARS was dramatic and impactful. Overall, the co-ordinated scientific response to SARS was monumental. SARS, like the H1N1 influenza pandemic of recent, has humbled the medical and scientific communities but has equally provided the catalyst to stimulate emergency preparedness for the next regional or global infectious pandemic.

Food For Thought

1. Review the current status of the epidemiology of West Nile virus and similar viruses.
2. What evidence is there for airborne spread of MRSA?
3. An outbreak has occurred in your community in which nearly 300 people have been infected by a diarrheal pathogen over the course of one week. What strategies might be used to both inform and calm the public?
4. How does one differentiate 'emerging infectious diseases' from 're-emerging infectious diseases'?
5. Why the panic over SARS-CoV? Was it truly a new virus?

Supplemental Reading

Cimolai N. MRSA and the environment: implications for comprehensive control measures. *European Journal of Clinical Microbiology and Infectious Diseases* Vol. 27: pp.481-493 (2008).
- an example of how the inanimate context may have a role in maintaining the germ

Cimolai N. The role of healthcare personnel in the maintenance and spread of methicillin-resistant *Staphylococcus aureus*. *Journal of Infection and Public Health* Vol. 1: pages 78-100 (2008).
- an example of how healthcare personnel may have a role in transmission

240

Cimolai N. Methicillin-resistant *Staphylococcus aureus* (MRSA) in Canada: historical perspective and lessons learned. *Canadian Journal of Microbiology* Vol. 56: pages 89-120 (2010).
- lessons learned here translate into learning everywhere else

DeSalle R – ed. *Epidemic! The World of Infectious Disease*. New York, NY:The New Press, 1999.
- a short but enjoyable overview

Hui DS, Chan PK. Severe acute respiratory syndrome and coronavirus. *Infectious Disease Clinics of North America* Vol. 24: pages 619-638 (2010).
- a good summation of the SARS epidemic

Kahn JS. The widening scope of coronaviruses. *Current Opinion in Pediatrics* Vol. 18: pages 42-47 (2006).
- how the understanding of SARS opened new doors

Ryan F. *Virus X: Tracking the New Killer Plagues Out of the Present and Into the Future*. New York, NY:Little, Brown, and Co., 1997.
- fun and light reading; think of how emerging infections have impacted the world since this book was written

Scheld WM, Hammer SM, Hughes JM – eds. *Emerging Infections* – Series. Washington, DC:ASM Press, 2008 (Volume 8).
- yearly reports of emerging infections from scientific and medical congress

"Against the disease of writing, one must take special precautions,
since it is a dangerous and contagious disease."
Peter Abelhard, 1079-1142
Letter 8, Abelhard to Heloise

XVIII. Infection Control Glossary

abscess – an infected cavity among tissue which is filled with pus and the products of infection as well as the infectious agents.

acid-fast stain - see Ziehl-Neelsen stain.

active immunization - immunization accomplished with the use of a vaccination.

active surveillance – generally refers to processes in active health care institutions which monitor infection on an ongoing basis and proactively rather than in a retrospective fashion.

acute care – health care settings where active patient care occurs and the level of illness acuity is high.

aerobic – can grow in the presence of oxygen.

aerosol – spread through air as small particles.

agar - a solid growth medium for bacterium isolation in the laboratory.

agglutination – the physical clumping which may be seen when antigen-antibody reactions occur. It may be used to detect antigen or antibody depending on the configuration of the assay.

AIDS – acquired immunodeficiency syndrome.

aldehyde – a chemical agent which is often used in decontaminating medical supplies.

ambulatory care – patient care in a context where patients are mobile and do not require admission to rooms with stay. For example, care given in a health care clinic is ambulatory care.

aminoglycosides – a class of antibiotics with unique structure and which are structurally and functionally much different from penicillin-like antibiotics. These antibiotics act in the bacterial cell at the level of protein synthesis.

anaerobic – grows mainly or only in the absence of oxygen.

anthrax – infection caused by *Bacillus anthracis*. Mainly a zoonosis, but recent notoriety has raised concern with regard to its use as a biological weapon.

antibiogram – the pattern of antibiotic susceptibilities and resistances.

antibiotic – a natural or synthetic substance that provides antimicrobial activity. In lay terms, this often refers to substances that are antibacterial.

antibiotic-associated diarrhea - a gastrointestinal illness which arises as a consequence of the disruption of the normal flora of the bowel during antibiotic treatment. A key culprit in this disease is *Clostridium difficile*.

antibody – a protein produced by specific cells (B cells) which is active in immunity. The protein effectively latches on to the foreign substance.

antifungal – activity against fungi.

antigen - structure capable of inducing an immune response.

antimicrobial – activity against microbes, although most people often interchange this with antibiotic.

antiparasitic – activity against parasites.

antiseptic – a chemical which reduces the risk for bacterial infection when applied to the body. For example, antiseptic soaps are used to reduce the contamination of skin in preparation for surgery.

antisepsis – a state in which antiseptic use has been effective.

antiserum - a component of blood that contains antibody to a microbe and which is usually produced by immunization of the source individual or animal.

antiviral – activity against viruses.

arthropod – type of insect.

asepsis – a state in which infectious risk has been reduced or entirely remove.

attenuated – altered or changed. For example, an attentuated virus vaccine may contain viable virus, but it has been changed in the laboratory to make it less likely to cause its usual disease.

autoclave - a sterilizing chamber in which the killing effect on germs is achieved with the combination of heat and pressure.

auto-infection – infection caused by microbes which are normally part of the usual microbial flora.

AZT – the old abbreviation for the anti-HIV antiviral agent known as zidovudine. It was historically one of the first and most effective of anti-HIV agents.

B cells - a lineage of mononuclear white blood cell in the body which is capable of producing antibody.

bacillus – the morphology of a bacterium that is elongated.

bacteremia – blood-borne infection.

bacterial vaginosis – a condition of the female vagina in which there is a highly abnormal composition of the vaginal flora and in which the patient usually suffers from a vaginal discharge and odour.

bactericidal – ability to kill bacteria.

bacteriocin typing – a fingerprinting method for some bacteria whereby strains of a species will variably produce antibacterial products.

bacteriology - the study of bacteria.

bacteriophage – a bacterial virus.

bacteriostatic - capable of inhibiting a bacterium.

bacterium – a procaryotic micro-organism that is usually capable of self-replication and which has a cell membrane.

BCG – an abbreviation for Bacille Calmette-Guérin which is an attenuated bovine mycobacterium. It is used as a vaccine to diminish the likelihood of developing tuberculosis.

beta-lactam – a type of antibiotic which resembles penicillins or cephalosporins, and which possesses a chemical beta-lactam ring (see Chapter IX).

beta-lactamase – an enzyme which is capable of destroying the beta-lactam ring of a beta-lactam antibiotic.

binary fission – the mechanism by which a microbe divides and replicates by way of splitting into two.

bioactivity – biological action.

biofilm – a surface covering which is composed of the microbe and its extracellular product in addition to some human substances. These may coat intravenous devices over a period of time.

biohazard - a biological substance, living or not, which poses a risk to human health.

biomass - total weight, volume, or number of microbial organisms.

biotyping – a fingerprinting method for bacterial strain differentiation which depends on variation among biochemical abilities among bacteria.

blood-brain barrier - the limiting and dividing tissue that separates the blood space from the cerebrospinal fluid space.

Body Substance Precautions – the term used to describe a process by which acquisition of infection is diminished but with emphasis on the blood and body fluid borne viral pathogens (see Chapter VI).

botulism – a neurological illness caused by the toxins of *Clostridium botulinum*.

brucellosis – a systemic infection caused by the *Brucella* bacteria.

candidiasis – a yeast infection caused by one of the *Candida* species. The most common cause is *C. albicans*. Infection may be superficial (e.g., diaper rash, thrush, vaginitis) or systemic.

capnophile – a bacterium that grows well in the presence of carbon dioxide.

carriage – the presence of an infectious agent at a body site for a long period of time whereby disease is not necessarily caused. The person or animal which maintains the germ is called a 'carrier'.

cell-mediated immunity – immunity which is dependent on the actions of immune cells that are not primarily antibody producing nor mainly phagocytic.

central venous line – an intravenous tubing that goes into a large vein. The large vein access is chosen because the infusion may be of large volume or because the infusion needs to be instantly mixed with a large volume of blood in the body. This form of venous access can remain secure for a much longer time than usual peripheral vein access.

cephalosporin – a chemical modification of the penicillin antibiotic and essentially a new antibiotic class. The mechanism of action is similar to penicillin(s) (see Chapter IX).

cervicitis – inflammation of the cervix. Infectious causes include *Chlamydia trachomatis* and *Neisseria gonorrhoeae*.

chicken pox – the infection caused after first contact with varicella-zoster virus. It is mainly a skin affliction, but systemic disease can also occur especially in patients with suppressed immune systems.

cholera – infection caused by *Vibrio cholerae*. The illness is a profuse watery diarrhea.

cirrhosis – end-stage scarring of the liver caused by long-standing inflammation.

clonality – the similarity among isolates suggesting a common clone.

clone – a common group of isolates from species which may have been derived directly from one another. It may also indicate a direct copy of another microbe.

coagulase negative staphylococci – staphylococci which do not have the coagulase enzyme. These generally include all those staphylcocci that are not *Staphylococcus aureus*.

coccus – the spherical or oval form of a bacterium.

coliform – the appearance of a Gram negative rod from Gram staining which is typical of bacteria from the *Enterobacteriaceae* family.

colonization – the natural presence of a microbe, most commonly a bacterium, among the normal flora of the body.

colony (of bacteria) – the appearance of the growth of isolated bacteria on laboratory agar media.

commensal – part of the normal microbial flora at a given body site.

communicable disease control – the public health aspects of identifying infection and preventing its spread.

community-acquired infection - an infection acquired in the general public domain and not from within a medical institution.

complement – a normal occuring set of proteins in the body which in part may have some immune functions. These are located circulating in blood.

complement fixation test – a serological test for the determination of antibody which relies on indirect detection via complement fixation (see Chapter IV).

congenital infection – infection of the fetus.

conjugation - a form of genetic transfer from bacterium to bacterium.

conjunctivitis – inflammation of the lining of the external eye. It may occur as a consequence of infection.

conjugate vaccine – a vaccine which is produced by the combination of two or more separate antigens. The union is purposeful so that the immune response to one antigen enhances the immune response to the other antigen.

contact tracing – the act of tracing for contacts of an infectious disease.

contagion - a burden of germs capable of causing infection.

cost-benefit ratio – a comparison of costs and then benefits of a medical process or manoeuvre. The ratio is a figurative assessment of the comparative aspects of this investigation.

cross-infection – an infection which has been transmitted from one patient to the next.

cryptosporidiosis – disease caused by the parasite *Cryptosporidium*. It is manifest as a diarrheal illness.

culture – the growth of a microbe under laboratory conditions.

cytokine – a chemical, usually protein, that is secreted by a human cell in response to various processes including infection and which activates or modulates other cells and bodily functions.

cytoplasm – the interior of a cell.

cytotoxin - a toxin which is capable of causing cellular disease and possibly including cell death.

decontamination – the eradication or reduction of infectious agents from their sources.

decubitus – lying down or against in a certain position. In reference to decubitus ulcers (also known as pressure sores), an area of ulceration or denudation of skin occurs in response to prolonged pressure in a given position and environment.

demographics – the study of people, their geographic distribution, and their environment.

dengue fever – a viral illness which is transmitted by mosquitoes. It is caused by the dengue fever virus and has geographic limitations.

detergent – a chemical that has solubilizing effects especially for fatty substances.

dialysis - also known as the artificial kidney. A process in which the body is cleansed from substances that would otherwise be the function of the normal kidneys.

diphtheria – the infection caused by *Corynebacterium diphtheriae*. The illness often begins with a severe sore throat, and toxin absorption may then lead to systemic effects.

discriminatory power – a measure of the degree by which strains of a bacterium may be differentiated with the use of a fingerprinting technique.

disinfection – the removal and diminution of infectious agents on inanimate objects.

DNA – deoxyribonucleic acid. The major biochemical structure which acts as the genetic code for life in most higher microbes and other life forms.

dose-response - the outcome of an infection or treatment which is dependent on the quantity of the input.

ectoparasite – a parasite which causes infection outside of the body (e.g., lice).

encephalitis – an infection of the brain tissue.

enterococci – a common term for Gram positive bacteria of the *Enterococcus* genus. These are very common in the intestinal tract, hence the 'entero-'.

enterohemorrhagic – capable of inducing bleeding in the gastrointestinal system. This term is often used in the context of verotoxigenic *E. coli* which may cause a bloody diarrhea, but perhaps it is a misnomer because there are other bacteria which are capable of causing bloody diarrhea in some patients (e.g., *Salmonella, Shigella, Yersinia enterocolitica, Campylobacter*).

enterotoxin - a bacterial toxin which is capable of causing disease in the intestinal tract.

enzyme – a protein which is able to make a biochemical conversion.

enzyme immunoassay – a stepwise procedure which is used in the laboratory to detect antigen or antibody depending on the configuration of the assay. The steps in this test make use of antibodies and enzyme labels.

epidemic – an increase in the frequency of an infection in a given context above the baseline norm. Generally the term is used to describe a great increase in such frequency and especially with reference to a commonality of source.

epidemiology – the scientific study of disease spread and presence.

eosinophil - a variation of polymorphonuclear cells that is commonly associated with allergic reactions and which is occasionally increased in the circulating blood during parasite infections.

ethylene oxide – a chemical gas which is used as a type of sterilizing agent and which does not require elevated temperature.

eukaryote - more advanced form than prokaryotes. A eukaryote has a nucleus and a nuclear membrane in its cells. Eukaryotes include parasites, fungi, and higher orders of living forms like plants and animals.

Family - a stratum of taxonomy ranked above Genus. The Family includes a larger cluster of similarly-structured organisms.

filariasis - systemic infection caused by specific small parasites which is geographically limited. One phase of the parasite causes bloodborne infestation.

fimbriae – short proteinaceous projections from the surface of bacteria which serve as either attachment factors or as tubules for bacteria to interchange genetic material.

fingerprinting (bacterial) – synonymous with 'typing' which indicates a method which is used to show similarity or dissimilarity among bacterial isolates.

flagellum – a protein complex whip-like organelle of a bacterium that provides for motility.

fluorescence microscopy - a form of diagnostic microscopy in which fluorescent tags are used to identify a microbe or an immune response to a microbe. This requires a sophisticated type of microscope.

food poisoning - usually a short incubation and short-lived illness caused by preformed toxin of particular microbes in food. Sometimes more loosely used as a term to denote any infection acquired from a food.

fungicidal – ability to kill fungi.

fungistatic – ability to inhibit fungi.

fungus – a eukaryotic microbe which is common in the environment. It may exist as yeast or mold form.

gastroenteritis – an infection of the gastrointestinal tract and most commonly used to denote a diarrheal illness.

genetic detection - used to describe the diagnosis of infection by the direct detection of the infecting microbe's DNA or RNA in the clinical sample.

genome – the genetic material which makes up the basis for microbial existence, function, and replication.

genus – a taxonomic term used to ascribe grouping between the family and species levels. Attribution to a particular genus is a function of the degree of genetic relatedness. For example, in *Escherichia coli*, 'Escherichia' denotes the genus name.

germ – synonymous with 'microbe'.

germ theory - the thesis that microbes were the cause of infection.

germicidal – a chemical agent which is capable of destroying germs.

germistatic - capable of inhibiting the germ.

giardiasis – infection caused by the parasite *Giardia*. This usually is a diarrheal illness only.

glycopeptide – a class of antibiotic which includes vancomycin and like agents. These are cell wall active agents with a different site of action in comparison to penicillin(s).

gonorrhea – infection caused by *Neisseria gonorrhoeae*. This is usually a genital infection. It is a sexually transmitted disease except for direct acquisition by a newborn from an infected mother.

gowning – the act of wearing a gown for preventing contact with an infectious agent.

Gram stain – a popular and long-standing technique for staining bacteria so that they may be seen under the microscope. Bacteria are Gram positive (purple), Gram negative (red), or non-stainable.

HBIG – a popular abbreviation for hepatitis B immune globulin. A purified source of human antibody which is active against hepatitis B.

hemophiliac – a patient who has an inherited disorder which leads to improper blood clotting. The defiency occurs in one or more coagulation proteins.

hemorrhagic fever – an illness due to some arboviruses (e.g., Ebola virus) which is characterized by a coagulation disorder during the course of the illness.

hepatitis - liver inflammation which can be caused by infection or other noxious agent.

HIV – abbeviation for human immunodeficiency virus which is the cause of AIDS.

home care – patient care which is delivered to the home and usually for a chronic condition or a condition where prolonged care and follow-up are needed.

humoral immune response - the type of immune response which leads to antibody production.

HUS – abbreviation for hemolytic uremic syndrome. The most common infectious cause is verotoxigenic *Escherichia coli*.

hydrogen peroxide – a chemical disinfectant and antiseptic that is commonly available over-the-counter. It is often used as a home remedy for cleaning minor wounds. The chemical composition is purely of hydrogen and oxygen. Oxygen radicals are generated.

hygiene – a science of health in general.

hyphae – strands of fungal molds.

iatrogenic - an illness caused by the caregiver (e.g., an iatrogenic infection is that which occurred due to a medical procedure).

immunoblotting – a serological technique which is used for antibody detection. The method is often referred to as a confirmatory test because reactivity of antibody to a specific antigen can be definitively visualized.

immunodeficiency – an impairment in or lack of usual immunity.

immunogen – a substance which evokes an antibody response to itself. Occasionally, this term may be used in place of 'vaccine'.

immunoglobulin – synonymous with 'antibody'.

immunology – the science of the immune system.

incidence – in regard to infections, it is the number of new episodes which have occurred in a given unit time.

incubation period – the time between new acquisition of the infectious agent and the onset of the infection.

index case – the first case of the given infection that acts as the source for other infections.

infection – a consequence of host-microbial interaction in which favour towards the microbe tips the balance for disease.

infection control committee – a committee within a health care setting structure which is responsible largely for devising the policy and procedure for infection control.

infection control manual – a text which details the policies and procedures for infection control in a health care institution.

infection control service - the sector of the medical institution that is specifically charged with the implementation of infection control policy and procedure.

influenza – a generalized illness caused by influenza viruses.

infusate – the liquid which is infused through an intravenous device.

insecticide – an agent which is capable of inhibiting or killing insects.

insertion sequences – repeat elements in a bacterial genome.

intravenous – given via the vein.

iodophor – a chemical compound that liberates iodine during its interaction with inanimate objects or host tissue.

isolate – a culture isolation of a microbe in the laboratory.

isolation – in the context of bacteriology, it refers to the culture process. In regards to infection control, it refers to quarantine.

Legionnaire's disease – illness caused by *Legionella* species. Usually this is manifest as respiratory illness.

leprosy – disease caused by *Mycobacterium leprae*. The disease is a disfiguring one when the skin is involved, but the infection can be systemic.

lice – ectoparasites that cause skin irritation and which may act as vectors for some bacterial infections.

life cycle - the pattern of growth of an organism from genesis to maturity and including all of the intermediate stages.

live-attenuated vaccine - a vaccine which is based on the laboratory changes in a microbe which allow it to be alive while not simultaneously being able to cause infection.

Lyme disease – infection caused by specific *Borrelia* species (e.g., *Borrelia burgdorferi*). The disease may be manifest as a skin eruption or may progress to involve heart, joints, and central nervous system.

lymphocyte – a type of white blood cell. Some lymphocytes are capable of producing antibodies, while others participate in cell-mediated immunity.

M cells - a specific cell type that lines the mucosa (e.g., gastrointestinal tract) and is capable of assisting in the development of local immunity.

macrophage - a large immune cell which has phagocytic and immune processing functions.

malaria – infection caused by *Plasmodium* species. The infection is acquired by a mosquito bite, and it is a blood-borne infection with some phases in the liver. Its acquisition is geographically determined.

Mantoux test – a skin test for tuberculosis. A purified protein derivative is injected under the skin. If a particularly sized red and indurated reaction occurs over 2-3 days at the skin site, the test may be regarded as evidence for current or past infection by *Mycobacterium tuberculosis*.

measles – infection caused by the measles virus. It includes a respiratory infection and rash. It is also known as rubeola or red measles.

membrane – a lipid (fatty) bilayer which surrounds the cytoplasm of bacteria and mammalian cells.

meningitis – infection of the linings which cover the brain and spinal cord.

meningococci – a common term for *Neisseria meningitidis*.

microaerophile – a bacterium that prefers a growth environment that has reduced quantities of oxygen.

microbe – a microscopic infectious agent.

microscopy – the science of the use of the microscope.

mold – a filamentous form of fungus, in contrast to yeast which are unicellular.

molecular biology - the field of biology in which the study focuses on molecular events, especially those that relate to genetic reproduction, structure, and function.

mononucleosis - a clinical illness of fever, sore throat, and general malaise which is caused by the Epstein-Barr virus. The name highlights the common finding of mononuclear white blood cells in large numbers in the blood.

MRSA – an abbreviation for methicillin-resistant *Staphylococcal aureus*.

mucous membrane – the barrier lining of the mouth, intestines, and female genital tract.

multi-resistant bacteria – bacteria which are resistant to several key antibiotics at one time.

mumps – a viral infection caused by mumps virus. Although classically a febrile illness that is accompanied by enlarged salivary glands of the face, the virus can cause a systemic illness as well.

mutation – a spontaneous change in genetic material.

mycology - the study of fungi.

necrotizing fasciitis – a deep-seated infection of muscle and connective tissue. In its worst form, it may cause a progressive death of tissue that may not respond to antibacterial antibiotics as bacterial enzymes continue to damage the area.

needlestick injury – an injury suffered as a consequence of percutaneous exposure to a sharp object.

non-A, non-B hepatitis - historical term used to denote a likely infectious hepatitis that was not caused by either hepatitis A or hepatitis B. Many of the causations proved to be hepatitis C virus.

normal flora - the usual microbes that are associated with different body sites in the nondiseased state.

nosocomial – occurring within a hospital.

opportunistic – causing infection at an 'opportune' time when the host is compromised for whatever reason (e.g., immune compromise).

opsonin – factors (e.g., proteins) which promote phagocytosis.

otitis media – infection of the middle ear. It is a common childhood infection.

outbreak – occurrence of more than the usual anticipated number of infections given the known background endemic frequency.

pandemic – an epidemic affecting a much larger region. For example, one could have an epidemic of infection among all the residents of a nursing home, but one also have a pandemic affecting most continents with the same illness (e.g., influenza).

parasite – in the context of proper nomenclature, a parasite is of a unique group of eukaryotic living forms which are capable of causing infection. In the discussion of the host-parasite relationship, we then may use the word to describe any cause of infection.

parasitology - the study of parasites.

parenteral – administered by a route other than by mouth (e.g., a parenteral antibiotic may be given by intravenous) (e.g., a parenteral vaccine may be given by injection).

passive immunization - the recipient achieves immune protection by way of receiving an antiserum that has been produced in another immunized or immune subject.

passive surveillance – a review which is based on the provision of data from the active care site and which may be retrospective, rather than by an active perusal and search for the same (i.e., contrast with active surveillance).

pasteurization – a disinfection method that uses high heat for a given period of time but which is less than boiling temperature (e.g., 70°C for 20 minutes).

pathogenic - capable of causing disease.

PCR – an abbreviation for polymerase chain reaction. It is an amplification process which allows for the massive reproduction of short sequences of DNA or RNA.

penicillin – first of a class of antibiotics. The original penicillin was a natural product, but newer versions have arisen from chemical modifications of the basic structure. The antibiotic and similar ones have a beta-lactam nucleus. They act on the cell wall synthesis pathways.

penicillinase – an enzyme that is capable of destroying penicillin.

pertussis – the respiratory illness caused by *Bordetella pertussis*. It is also known as whooping cough.

phage typing – a bacterial fingerprinting method in which differences in bacteria are assessed by variable susceptibility to a pool of bacterial viruses.

phagocyte – a human cell that is capable of engulfing and digesting a microbial pathogen.

phagocytosis – the process by which a phagocytic cell destroys a pathogen. This involves uptake into the human cell and then subsequent destruction.

phenolic – a chemical agent class which is commonly used in household and hospital disinfectants. The basic structure of these is in common with 'phenol'.

pilus – plural as 'pili' and synonymous with fimbriae.

plague – the infection caused by the bacterium *Yersinia pestis*.

plasmid – circular piece of DNA among bacteria that exists in addition to the long chromosome. Some rare bacteria may have linear plasmids.

pneumococci – common term for *Streptococcus pneumoniae*.

pneumonia – an infection of the lung. It may be very focussed or throughout the lung.

polio – disease caused by the polio virus. The illness is a neurological disease, and it is preventable by vaccination.

polymyxin – a unique antibiotic class which is used only as a topical agent. This group of antibiotics is capable of poking holes in the membranes of select bacterial cells.

polymorphonuclear cell – when viewed under the microscope, this type of white blood cell has multiple lobes to its nucleus. There are several types of such cells. The most common is a phagocytic cell and a major component of pus.

polysaccharide – a complex sugar molecule. It is the basis for bacterial capsules.

potable water – drinkable water for general consumption.

prevalence – in reference to infections, it refers to the number of such infections which exist at any one point in time.

prion – an abbreviation for 'protein infectious agent'. The agent of 'Mad Cow Disease', it is believed that the transmissible agent is a protein rather than either virus, bacterium, fungus, or parasite.

procaryote – primitive form of life such as viruses or bacteria which do not possess mitochondria or do not divide by mitosis.

prophylaxis – infection prevention usually given in the form of vaccine or antibiotic.

protozoa – consist mainly of unicellular forms of parasites (e.g., malaria parasites).

pseudomonad – Gram negative bacteria that structurally and biochemically resemble *Pseudomonas* species.

public health – the science of preserving the health of the public at large on a population basis.

pus – the collection of white blood cells and other materials that result from infection in response to active infection. Pus looks usually yellow or green.

Q fever – a systemic illness caused by the bacterial agent *Coxiella burnetii*.

quarantine – isolation procedures for a patients with a given infection.

quaternary ammonium compounds - a group of chemicals which are commonly used for disinfection. They are commonly referred to a 'quats'.

quinolone – a class of antibiotic with unique structure and function. These agents interact with elements of genomic synthesis. Examples of this group include norfloxacin and ciprofloxacin.

rabies – the disease caused by rabies virus. It is transmitted from animals, and the illness is a neurological one with a long incubation period.

radioimmunoassay – an immunological technique for the detection of antigen or antibody, and which uses radio-isotopes as a marker.

receptor – the attachment site for an infectious agent on the host tissue or cells.

relapsing fever - a cyclical fever pattern caused by particular *Borrelia* species which appear in the bloodstream.

reportable disease - in the context of infection, a communicable disease for which there is legislated mandate to report to public health authorities.

reservoir – the source for an infectious agent.

risk factor – a factor or attribute that is associated with increased risk for a given disease (e.g., being a health care worker is an increased risk for some infections due to increased exposure).

risk management – the recognition, management, and prevention of risk factors for disease.

RNA – ribonucleic acid. A form of genetic material. For viruses, this may be the main genetic code. For higher forms of living forms, DNA is more often the main genetic code, and RNA acts as an intermediary form which converts the code of DNA into a workable product (e.g., protein).

roseola - infection of infants caused by a member of the human herpesviruses. It is characteristic in that there is a several day occurrence of high fever followed by a flat red rash after the fever subsides.

rubella – a systemic illness caused by rubella virus. This infection is often referred to as 'German measles'. It is currently prevented by vaccination.

salmonellosis – infection caused by *Salmonella* species. These are most often diarrheal illnesses.

sanitizer – a common low grade household disinfectant.

SARS - severe acute respiratory syndrome which is caused by the human coronavirus variant.

scabies – a dermatological illness caused by the ectoparasite called *Sarcoptes scabeii*.

schistosomiasis – a systemic infection due to the parasites called 'schistosomes'. The infection is confined to geographic areas that support schistosome transmission.

sepsis – the presence of bacteria in blood or tissue and causing active illness.

seroconversion - the demonstration that a new humoral immune response has taken place which is directed to a particular germ.

serodiagnosis - laboratory diagnosis which is facilitated by the discovery of new humoral immune responses to a germ, which implies the recent onset of infection by that same germ.

serology – a diagnostic method in which infection is determined by the detection of microbe-specific antibodies.

serotyping – a method of bacterial fingerprinting which depends on the unique attributes of surface antigens as determined serologically. The method is currently used to separate *Salmonella* isolates.

sharps container – a safety deposit box for the discard of sharp medical supplies (e.g., needles).

sharps injury – an injury suffered as a consequence of percutaneous breach with a sharp medical instrument.

shigellosis – infection caused by *Shigella* species. This is almost always a diarrheal illness.

sinusitis – infection of the sinus cavities of the head.

smallpox – disease caused by smallpox virus. Now eradicated from the world through the efforts of vaccination, it was once a dreaded illness and major killer.

species – a unique biological division which depends on the similarity of genetic material to other living forms. The division is a more specific category than the genus designation.

spirochete – a spiral form of bacterium. Such bacteria include very few, but most notable are *Treponema pallidum* and *Borrelia* species.

spore – a sessile or dormant form of a bacterium or fungus. Bacterial spores are very resistant to decontaminating agents.

sporicidal – capable of killing spores.

Standard Precautions – a new designation for the 'standard' approach to policies and procedures for infection control (see Chapter VI).

staphylococci ("staph") – Gram positive cocci in clusters. These include *S. aureus* and coagulase-negative staphylococci.

sterile supply service – that area of a health care institution that provides clean materials for medical use and reuse. For example, the sterile supply area of the hospital may be responsible for cleaning and supply of medical surgical instruments to the operating room suites.

sterilant – an agent that provides sterility.

sterilization – the process by which an object is rendered free of any living form or any form that may develop into a living form.

strain – a unique version of a bacterial species.

sulpha antibiotics (sulpha drugs) - a unique class of antibiotics more technically known as sulphonamides. These are mainly of antibacterial use. This group was one of the earliest discovered for clinical use.

superbug - a lay term used to denote a bacterium with multiple antibiotic resistances. Historically used to imply MRSA.

susceptibility testing – the process of determining whether a microbe can be killed or inhibited by antibiotics by means of a laboratory assessment.

symbiosis - the mutual co-existence of two living organisms in which there is a benefit for both.

syphilis – infection cause by *Treponema pallidum*. It is a sexually transmitted disease except for congenital infection. It may be localized to the genital area or become systemic.

T cells - a lineage of mononuclear white blood cells in the body which have a role in the control of infection and in the modulation of the immune response.

tapeworm - a segmented parasite capable of living in the intestinal tract.

taxonomy – the science of microbial classification in our context.

tetanus – disease caused by the bacterium *Clostridium tetani*. The illness is a neurological one and is caused by bacterial toxin.

toxic shock syndrome – a cluster of disease manifestations which are attributable to a toxin from some *Staphylococcus aureus* isolates. In the advanced illness, patients may have 'shock' which is circulatory collapse.

toxigenic - capable of producing a toxin.

toxin – an agent, often protein, which is secreted by a bacterium and which may have some directed physiological effect on host tissue.

toxoid – an inactivated toxin. A toxoid may be safely used in a vaccine since the toxin activity is obliterated.

transformation - the uptake of genetic material from the environment by a bacterium which may then change the bacterium's genetic material and capability.

transmission – the transfer of infection.

transposon – a 'jumping gene'. A gene which has the ability to be mobilized from one part of the genome to the other. This 'jumping' may occur from one part of the chromosome to another, or from plasmid to chromosome or vice versa.

trichinosis – disease caused by the parasite *Trichinella*. After ingestion of live larvae from a food source, the parasite enters the body where it causes a massive allergic reaction.

tropism – has an affinity for.

tuberculosis – an infection caused by *Mycobacterium tuberculosis*. Although most often thought of as a lung infection, the bacterium may spread to almost any other body site.

typeability – the likelihood that a typing method will discriminate among isolates when variation is actually present. Essentially describes the efficiency of a typing method to do its intended work.

typing – synonymous with 'fingerprinting'. A method for differentiating isolates.

typhoid fever – infection caused by *Salmonella typhi*. It is a systemic illness in contract to most other salmonelloses which are diarrheal illnesses. It is mainly an infection which is acquired in areas with poor sanitation.

Universal Precautions – a designation given to the collection of policies and procedures which arose in the 1980s as a consequence of the need to address the potential for the acquisition of blood-borne viruses from various materials (see Chapter VI).

urinary tract infection – an infection of the urinary tract but most commonly referring to bladder infections or infections of the kidney.

vaccine – a material which is from a microbe and which is administered to the host in order to stimulate protective immunity.

vaginitis – an inflammatory process of the female vagina. In the context of infection, the common causes include yeast, *Trichomonas vaginalis* (a parasite), bacterial vaginosis, and herpes simplex.

vector – the intermediate which acts to transmit the cause of an infection from one source to another source. A vector can be living or inanimate.

venipuncture – the process of collecting blood through a needle and container (e.g., syringe).

ventilation – air circulation in a given environment. In the setting of a hospital, 'positive pressure' ventilation forces air into the room from a duct and the escaping air must exit the room, whereas in 'negative pressure' ventilation, air is drawn into the room from the outside and is then exhausted through a vent to the outside.

viridans streptococci - are usually normal flora streptococci of the mouth and intestinal tract which are also capable of causing infection.

virology - the study of viruses.

virucidal – the ability to kill a virus.

virulence – the varying ability for a microbe to cause disease. 'Virulence factors' (or virulence determinants) are those components of a microbe that facilitate or cause infection.

virustatic – the ability to inhibit a virus.

virus – a procaryotic microbe that depends on the host cell for replication. Viruses are intracellular pathogens. They lack self-produced membranes. They have either DNA or RNA as the main genetic material.

VISA – vancomycin intermediately-susceptible *Staphylococcus aureus*.

VRE – vancomycin-resistant enterococci.

VZIG – varicella-zoster immune globulin. Antibody from human sources which is used for the purposes of prophylaxis against varicella-zoster virus.

Western blotting – a laboratory method for separating proteins according to size and shape, and the subsequent transfer to a solid membrane support on which immunoblotting can be performed. The name commonly arises when one is discussing confirmatory serology for HIV infection.

whooping cough - the clinical respiratory illness caused by *Bordetella pertussis*.

wound – a physical result of direct trauma or surgical laceration to a skin site.

yeast – a unicellular form of fungus.

yellow fever – a systemic illness caused by yellow fever virus, which is an arbovirus. The 'yellow' refers to the jaundice which may occur when the liver has been sufficiently diseased.

yersiniosis – infection caused by *Yersinia enterocolitica*. Although mainly a diarrheal illness, some may include mainly severe abdominal pain which mimics appendicitis.

Ziehl-Neelsen stain - general unique stain used to detect mycobacteria in clinical specimens. Particularly used to diagnose tuberculosis. Also known as the acid-fast stain.

zoonosis – an infection acquired from animals either directly or indirectly.

zoster - synonymous with the clinical illness called 'shingles' and caused by a relapse of infection by the varicella zoster virus.

"Learn some, teach some,
Then learn some again."
　　　　　Nevio and Debra Cimolai
　　　　　Kitchen Table Talk, 2011

XIX. Profile of Medically Relevant Bacteria
(note: profile of published bacterial names can be found on the Internet at: http://www.bacteria.cict.fr/)

Name	category	associations
Abiotrophia species	Gram + coccus	streptococcus-like, uncommon cause of human infection, mainly blood-borne
Acholeplasma species	not Gram stained	commensal mycoplasma
Achromobacter species (some formerly *Alcaligenes*)	Gram – bacillus	rare infection, opportunistic, a pseudomonad
Acidominococcus species	Gram – coccus	anaerobic, rare cause of infection
Acidovorax (formerly a *Pseudomonas* species)	Gram – bacillus	rare infection, opportunistic, a pseudomonad
Acinetobacter species	Gram – bacillus	opportunists in human infection, from environmental sources, a pseudomonad
Actinobacillus species	Gram – coccobacillus	uncommon causes of wound, respiratory, and blood infection, some species are of animal sources
Actinobaculum species	Gram + bacillus	rare cause of human infection
Actinomadura madurae	Gram variable	deep skin infections in tropical areas
Actinomyces israelii	Gram + bacillus	rare cause of chronic illness called actinomycosis, part of salivary flora
Actinomyces meyeri	Gram + bacillus	rare cause of infection, part of salivary flora
Actinomyces naeslundii	Gram + bacillus	rare cause of infection, part of salivary flora
Actinomyces neuii	Gram + bacillus	rare cause of human infection
Actinomyces odontolyticus	Gram + bacillus	rare cause of infection, part of salivary flora
Actinomyces radingae	Gram + bacillus	rare cause of human infection

Actinomyces turicensis	Gram + bacillus	rare cause of human infection
Actinomyces viscosus	Gram + bacillus	rare cause of infection, part of salivary flora
Advenella species	Gram – bacillus	rare opportunistic infections, a pseudomonad
Aerococcus species	Gram + coccus	infections like the coagulase-negative staphylococci but much less common
Aeromonas bestiarum	Gram – bacillus	coliform, rare isolate
Aeromonas caviae	Gram – bacillus	coliform, rare isolate
Aeromonas hydrophila	Gram – bacillus	wound infections, rare opportunist, putative causeof diarrhea, coliform
Aeromonas jandaei	Gram – bacillus	coliform, rare isolate
Aeromonas schubertii	Gram – bacillus	coliform, rare isolate
Aeromonas veronii	Gram – bacillus	coliform, rare isolate
Afipia felis	Gram – bacillus	once thought to be the cause of cat scratch disease, now a rare isolate without disease association
Aggregatibacter species	Gram– bacillus	rare cause of heart and soft tissue infection
Alcaligenes faecalis	Gram– bacillus	rare opportunistic infection, a pseudomonad
Alloiococcus otitidis	Gram + coccus	resembles the coagulase-negative staphylococci but has only been found in middle ear effusions although not necessarily as a definitive causative agent
Amycolata species	Gram variable	rare human infections
Anaerobiospirillum species	Gram – bacterium	anaerobe, rare cause of human infection
Anaerococcus species	Gram + coccus	anaerobe, associated with infection of bowel and other mucosa
Arcanobacterium bernardiae (formerly *Actinomyces*)	Gram + bacillus	rare cause of human infection
Arcanobacterium haemolyticum	Gram + bacillus	rare cause of sore throat and skin rash
Arcanobacterium pyogenes (formerly *Actinomyces*)	Gram + bacillus	rare cause of human infection
Arcobacter butzleri (formerly *Campylobacter butzleri*)	Gram – curved bacillus	uncommon isolate, cause of diarrhea
Arcobacter cryaerophilus	Gram – curved bacillus	uncommon isolate, cause of diarrhea

Arthrobacter species (formerly groups B1, B3)	Gram + bacillus	rare cause of human infection
Bacillus anthracis	Gram + bacillus	spore-forming, cause of anthrax
Bacillus brevis	Gram + bacillus	spore-forming, rare cause of human infection
Bacillus cereus	Gram + bacillus	spore-forming, food poisoning, rare other infections
Bacillus circulans	Gram + bacillus	spore-forming, rare cause of human infection
Bacillus coagulans	Gram + bacillus	spore-forming, rare cause of human infection
Bacillus licheniformis	Gram + bacillus	spore-forming, rare cause of human infection
Bacillus pumilus	Gram + bacillus	spore-forming, rare cause of human infection
Bacillus sphaericus	Gram + bacillus	spore-forming, rare cause of human infection
Bacillus subtilis	Gram + bacillus	spore-forming, rare cause of human infection
Bacillus thuringiensis	Gram + bacillus	spore-forming, rare cause of human infection, used in pesticides as a natural antagonist
Bacteroides fragilis	Gram − bacillus	anaerobic, common bowel flora
Bacteroides ovatus	Gram − bacillus	anaerobic, common bowel flora
Bacteroides thetaiotaomicron	Gram − bacillus	anaerobic, common bowel flora
Bacteroides ureolyticus	Gram − bacillus	anaerobic, associated with the mucosa
Bacteroides vulgatus	Gram − bacillus	anaerobic, common bowel flora
Balneatrix alpica	Gram − bacillus	rare infection, opportunistic, a pseudomonad
Bartonella bacilliformis	Gram − bacillus	cause of infection in specific areas of South America
Bartonella clarridgeiae	Gram − bacillus	uncommon cause of cat scratch disease
Bartonella elizabethae	Gram − bacillus	uncommon cause of cat scratch disease
Bartonella henselae	Gram − bacillus	common cause of cat scratch disease
Bartonella quintana	Gram − bacillus	cause of trench fever, louse transmitted

(formerly *Rickettsia quintana* and *Rochalimea quintana*)

Bartonella vinsonii	Gram – bacillus	canine source, very rare human infection
Bergeyella zoohelcum (formerly *Weeksella zoohelcum*)	Gram – bacillus	rare infection, opportunistic, a pseudomonad
Bifidobacterium species	Gram + bacillus	rare cause of human infection
Bilophila wadsworthia	Gram – bacillus	anaerobic, uncommon pathogen
Bordetella bronchiseptica	Gram – bacillus	rare human respiratory infection
Bordetella holmesii	Gram – bacillus	rare human pathogen
Bordetella parapertussis	Gram – coccobacillus	uncommon cause of a whooping cough-like illness
Bordetella pertussis	Gram – coccobacillus	cause of whooping cough
Bordetella trematum	Gram – bacillus	rare human pathogen
Borrelia afzelii	spirochete, not Gram stained	cause of Lyme disease, closely resembles *B. burgdorferi*
Borrelia burgdorferi	spirochete, not Gram stained	cause of Lyme disease
Borrelia duttonii	spirochete, not Gram stained	cause of relapsing fever
Borrelia garinii	spirochete, not Gram stained	cause of Lyme disease, closely resembles *B. burgdorferi*
Borrelia parkeri	spirochete, not Gram stained	cause of relapsing fever
Borrelia recurrentis	spirochete, not Gram stained	cause of relapsing fever
Borrelia turicatae	spirochete, not Gram stained	cause of relapsing fever
Brevibacillus species	Gram + bacillus	spore-forming, rare cause of human infection
Brevibacterium species	Gram + bacillus	rare cause of human infection
Brevundimonas species (formerly a *Pseudomonas*)	Gram – bacillus	rare infection, opportunistic, a pseudomonad
Brucella abortus	Gram – coccobacillus	cause of brucellosis, bovine source usually
Brucella canis	Gram – coccobacillus	cause of brucellosis, geographically limited
Brucella melitensis	Gram – coccobacillus	cause of brucellosis, geographically limited

Brucella suis	Gram – coccobacillus	cause of brucellosis, geographically limited
Budvicia species	Gram – bacillus	rare infection, uncommon isolate, coliform
Burkholderia cenocepacia	Gram – bacillus	highly resembles *Burkholderia cepacia*
Burkholderia cepacia (formerly a *Pseudomonas*)	Gram – bacillus	infects the lung in cystic fibrosis, several different species highly resemble it, rare causes of infection otherwise, a pseudomonad, environmental germ
Burkholderia dolosa	Gram – bacillus	highly resembles *Burkholderia cepacia*
Burkholderia multivorans	Gram – bacillus	highly resembles *Burkholderia cepacia*
Burkholderia pseudomallei	Gram – bacillus	causes melioidosis, geographically restricted
Burkholderia stabilis	Gram – bacillus	highly resembles *Burkholderia cepacia*
Burkholderia vietnamiensis	Gram – bacillus	highly resembles *Burkholderia cepacia*
Buttiauxella species	Gram – bacillus	rare infection, uncommon isolate, coliform
Butyrovibrio species	Gram – bacillus, may be curved	anaerobic, rare pathogen
Calymmatobacterium granulomatis (formerly *Donovania granulomatis*)	Gram – bacillus	rare cause of genital ulceration, sexually transmitted, difficult to culture
Campylobacter coli	Gram – curved bacillus	cause of diarrhea
Campylobacter concisus	Gram – curved bacillus	occasionally found in large bowel
Campylobacter curvus (formerly *Wolinella curva*)	Gram – curved bacillus	occasionally found in large bowel
Campylobacter fetus	Gram – curved bacillus	rare cause of invasive infection as an opportunist
Campylobacter gracilis (formerly *Bacteroides gracilis*)	Gram – curved bacillus	component of bowel flora
Campylobacter hyointestinalis	Gram – curved bacillus	uncommon isolate, animal source
Campylobacter jejuni	Gram – curved bacillus	cause of diarrhea
Campylobacter lari	Gram – curved bacillus	cause of diarrhea, uncommon isolate
Campylobacter rectus (formerly *Wolinella recta*)	Gram – curved bacillus	occasionally found in large bowel
Campylobacter sputorum	Gram – curved bacillus	occasionally found in large bowel
Campylobacter upsaliensis	Gram – curved bacillus	cause of diarrhea, uncommon isolate

Capnocytophaga species	Gram – coccobacillus	rare cause of infection
Cardiobacterium hominis	Gram – coccobacillus	rare cause of infection
Caulobacter species	Gram – bacillus	rare infection, opportunistic, a pseudomonad
Cedecea species	Gram – bacillus	rare infection, uncommon isolate, coliform
Cellulomonas species	Gram + bacillus	rare cause of human infection
Chlamydia pneumoniae	not Gram stained	respiratory pathogen, debated as a contributor to atherosclerosis
Chlamydia psittaci	not Gram stained	uncommon respiratory pathogen, from avians
Chlamydia trachomatis	not Gram stained	genital infection, rare respiratory infection, sexually transmitted disease
Chromobacterium violaceum	Gram – coccobacillus	rare cause of human infection
Chronoobacter sakazakii (formerly *Enterobacter sakazakii*)	Gram – bacillus	rare isolate, coliform
Chryseobacterium species (formerly *Flavobacterium*)	Gram – bacillus	rare infection, opportunistic, a pseudomonad
Citrobacter amalonaticus	Gram – bacillus	rare isolate, coliform
Citrobacter koseri (formerly *Citrobacter diversus*)	Gram – bacillus	common gut flora, opportunistic infection, coliform
Citrobacter farmeri	Gram – bacillus	rare isolate, coliform
Citrobacter freundii	Gram – bacillus	common gut flora, opportunistic infection, coliform
Citrobacter youngae	Gram – bacillus	rare isolate, coliform
Clostridium bifermentans	Gram + bacillus	spore-forming, part of bowel flora
Clostridium botulinum	Gram + bacillus	spore-forming, cause of botulism
Clostridium clostridioforme	Gram + bacillus	spore-forming, part of bowel flora
Clostridium difficile	Gram + bacillus	spore-forming, cause of antibiotic-associated diarrhea
Clostridium histolyticum	Gram + bacillus	spore-forming, part of bowel flora
Clostridium innocuum	Gram + bacillus	spore-forming, part of bowel flora
Clostridium novyi	Gram + bacillus	spore-forming, part of bowel flora
Clostridium perfringens	Gram + bacillus	spore-forming, part of bowel flora, most common cause of clostridial infection,

		abscesses, wound infection, gas gangrene
Clostridium ramosum	Gram + bacillus	spore-forming, part of bowel flora
Clostridium septicum	Gram + bacillus	spore-forming, part of bowel flora
Clostridium sordelli	Gram + bacillus	spore-forming, part of bowel flora
Clostridium sporogenes	Gram + bacillus	spore-forming, part of bowel flora
Clostridium tetani	Gram + bacillus	spore-forming, soil borne, cause of tetanus
Comamonas species	Gram – bacillus	rare infection, opportunistic, a pseudomonad
Coprococcus species	Gram + coccus	anaerobic, uncommon pathogen
Corynebacterium accolens (formerly CDC group 6)	Gram + bacillus	rare cause of infection
Corynebacterium afermentans	Gram + bacillus	rare cause of infection
Corynebacterium amycolatum (formerly CDC group F2)	Gram + bacillus	rare cause of infection
Corynebacterium auris	Gram + bacillus	rare cause of infection
Corynebacterium bovis	Gram + bacillus	rare cause of infection; usually bovine source
Corynebacterium confusum	Gram + bacillus	rare cause of infection
Corynebacterium coyleae	Gram + bacillus	rare cause of infection
Corynebacterium diphtheriae	Gram + bacillus	cause of diptheria, non-toxigenic forms may be carried on skin or in throat
Corynebacterium falsenii	Gram + bacillus	rare cause of infection
Corynebacterium glucuronolyticum	Gram + bacillus	rare cause of infection
Corynebacterium group F-1	Gram + bacillus	rare cause of infection, like corynebacteria
Corynebacterium group G	Gram + bacillus	rare cause of infection, like corynebacteria
Corynebacterium jeikeium	Gram + bacillus	rare cause of infection
Coryenbacterium kutscheri	Gram + bacillus	rare cause of infection
Corynebacterium macginleyi	Gram + bacillus	rare cause of infection
Corynebacterium matruchotii	Gram + bacillus	rare cause of infection
Corynebacterium minutissimum	Gram + bacillus	rare cause of infection, cause of skin condition known as erythrasma

Corynebacterium mucifaciens	Gram + bacillus	rare cause of infection
Corynebacterium propinquum (formerly ANF-3)	Gram + bacillus	rare cause of infection
Corynebacterium pseudodiphtheriticum	Gram + bacillus	rare cause of respiratory infection and others
Corynebacterium pseudotuberculosis	Gram + bacillus	rare cause of infection; mainly veterinary
Corynebacterium riegelii	Gram + bacillus	rare cause of infection
Corynebacterium simulans	Gram + bacillus	rare cause of infection
Corynebacterium singulare	Gram + bacillus	rare cause of infection
Corynebacterium striatum	Gram + bacillus	rare cause of infection
Corynebacterium sundvallense	Gram + bacillus	rare cause of infection
Corynebacterium thomssenii	Gram + bacillus	rare cause of infection
Corynebacterium ulcerans	Gram + bacillus	uncommon human infection, rare diphtheria-like illness and skin infection, animal source
Corynebacterium urealyticum (formerly group D2)	Gram + bacillus	uncommon cause of bladder infection
Corynebacterium xerosis	Gram + bacillus	rare cause of infection
Coxiella burnetii	not Gram stained	cause of Q fever
Cupriavidus gilardii (formerly an *Alcaligenes* and *Ralstonia gilardii*)	Gram – bacillus	rare opportunist, a pseudomonad
Cupriavidus pauculus (formerly CDC group IVc-2 and *Ralstonia paucula*)	Gram – bacillus	rare opportunist, a pseudomonad
Delftia acidovorans (formerly *Comamonas acidovorans* and *Pseudomonas acidovorans*)	Gram – bacillus	rare infection, opportunistic, a pseudomonad
Dermabacter species	Gram + bacillus	rare cause of human infection
Dermatophilus congolensis	Gram variable	rare skin infections, mainly an animal pathogen
Desulfomonas species	Gram – bacillus	anaerobic, rare pathogen
Desulfovibrio species	Gram – bacillus, can be curved	anaerobic, rare pathogen
Dialister species (formerly *Bacteroides*)	Gram – bacillus	anaerobic, rare pathogen
Dolosigranulum species	Gram + coccus	very rare infections

Dysgonomonas species	Gram – bacillus	rare cause of infection
Edwardsiella hoshinae	Gram – bacillus	rare isolate, coliform
Edwardsiella tarda	Gram – bacillus	uncommon isolate, putative cause of diarrhea, coliform
Ehrlichia canis	not Gram stained	cause of ehrlichiosis
Ehrlichia phagocytophila	not Gram stained	cause of ehrlichiosis
Ehrlichia sennetsu	not Gram stained	cause of ehrlichiosis, Sennetsu fever
Eikenella corrodens (formerly *Bacteroides corrodens*)	Gram – bacillus	uncommon cause of human infection, is of mucosal flora sources
Empedobacter brevis (formerly a *Flavobacterium*)	Gram – bacillus	rare infection, opportunistic, a pseudomonad
Enterobacter aerogenes	Gram – bacillus	common gut flora, opportunistic infection, coliform
Enterobacter cloacae	Gram – bacillus	common gut flora, opportunistic infection, coliform
Enterobacter gergoviae	Gram – bacillus	rare isolate, coliform
Enterococcus avium (*Enterococcus* genus formerly classified as *Streptococcus*)	Gram + coccus	a rare enterococcus, uncommon infections among humans
Enterococcus casseliflavus	Gram + coccus	a rare enterococcus, uncommon infections among humans
Enterococcus dispar	Gram + coccus	a rare enterococcus, uncommon infections among humans
Enterococcus durans	Gram + coccus	blood-borne infections, urinary tract infection, endocarditis, various others especially when related to breaks in the bowel mucosa
Enterococcus faecalis	Gram + coccus	blood-borne infections, urinary tract infection, endocarditis, various others especially when related to breaks in the bowel mucosa
Enterococcus faecium	Gram + coccus	blood-borne infections, urinary tract infection, endocarditis, various others especially when related to breaks in the bowel mucosa
Enterococcus gallinarum	Gram + coccus	a rare enterococcus, uncommon infections among humans

Enterococcus hirae	Gram + coccus	a rare enterococcus, uncommon infections among humans
Enterococcus malodoratus	Gram + coccus	a rare enterococcus, uncommon infections among humans
Enterococcus mundtii	Gram + coccus	a rare enterococcus, uncommon infections among humans
Enterococcus pseudoavium	Gram + coccus	a rare enterococcus, uncommon infections among humans
Enterococcus raffinosus	Gram + coccus	a rare enterococcus, uncommon infections among humans
Enterococcus saccharolyticus	Gram + coccus	a rare enterococcus, uncommon infections among humans
Erysipelothrix rhusiopathiae	Gram + bacillus	cause of erysipeloid, rare cause of blood-borne infections
Escherichia coli	Gram – bacillus	urinary tract infection, various forms of diarrhea, usually a common component of normal gut flora, opportunist, coliform
Escherichia fergusonii	Gram – bacillus	rare isolate, coliform
Escherichia hermannii	Gram – bacillus	rare isolate, coliform
Escherichia vulneris	Gram – bacillus	rare isolate, coliform
Eubacterium species	Gram + bacillus	rare cause of infection, common bowel flora
Ewingella americana	Gram – bacillus	rare isolate, coliform
Exiguobacterium species	Gram + bacillus	rare cause of human infection
Facklamia species	Gram + coccus	very rare cause of infection
Finegoldia magna (formerly *Peptostreptococcus magnus*)	Gram + coccus	anaerobic, associated with infection from bowel and other mucosal sources
Flavobacterium species	Gram – bacillus	rare infection, opportunistic, a pseudomonad
Francisella tularensis	Gram – coccobacillus	cause of tularemia, a zoonosis
Fusobacterium mortiferum	Gram – bacillus	anaerobic, part of mucosal flora
Fusobacterium necrophorum	Gram – bacillus	anaerobic, part of mucosal flora
Fusobacterium nucleatum	Gram – bacillus	anaerobic, part of mucosal flora
Fusobacterium varium	Gram – bacillus	anaerobic, part of mucosal flora
Gardnerella vaginalis	Gram variable	common component of vaginal flora, once thought to be the cause of bacterial

		vaginosis but no longer so
Gemella species	Gram + coccus	infections like the coagulase-negative staphylococci but much less common
Globicatella species	Gram + coccus	streptococcus-like, uncommon cause of human infection
Gordonia terrae	Gram variable	rare opportunist

Group A streptococci
  (see *Streptococcus pyogenes*)

Group B streptococci
  (see *Streptococcus agalactiae*)

Group C streptococci
  (see *Streptococcus dysgalactiae* subsp. *equisimilis* and *Streptococcus equi* subsp. *zooepidemicus*)

Group G streptococci
  (see *Streptococcus dysgalactiae* subsp. *equisimilis*)

Haemophilus aegyptius (formerly a biotpe of *Haemophilus influenzae*)	Gram – coccobacillus	conjunctivitis
Haemophilus aphrophilus	Gram – coccobacillus	rare cause of infection, mucosal commensal
Haemophilus ducreyi	Gram – coccobacillus	genital ulcers, a sexually transmitted pathogen
Haemophilus haemolyticus	Gram – coccobacillus	rare cause of infection
Haemophilus influenzae	Gram – coccobacillus	respiratory infection at all sites, invasive disease, meningitis, is a common component of usual respiratory flora
Haemophilus parahaemolyticus	Gram – coccobacillus	rare cause of infection, mucosal commensal
Haemophilus parainfluenzae	Gram – coccobacillus	occasional respiratory infection, a common component of usual respiratory flora
Haemophilus paraphrophilus	Gram – coccobacillus	rare cause of infection, mucosal commensal
Haemophilus segnis	Gram – coccobacillus	rare cause of infection
Hafnia alvei (formerly *Enterobacter alvei*)	Gram – bacillus	rare cause of infection, coliform, occasional component of normal gut flora
Helcococcus species	Gram + coccus	infections like the coagulase-negative staphylococci but much less common
Helicobacter canis	Gram – curved bacillus	rare isolate, cause of diarrhea
Helicobacter cinaedi (formerly *Campylobacter cinaedi*)	Gram – curved bacillus	rare isolate, cause of diarrhea, rare opportunist

Helicobacter fennelliae (formerly *Campylobacter fennelliae*)	Gram – curved bacillus	rare isolate, cause of diarrhea, rare opportunist
Helicobacter heilmannii (formerly *Gastrospirillum hominis*)	Gram – curved bacillus	rare isolate
Helicobacter pullorum	Gram – curves bacillus	rare isolate, cause of diarrhea
Helicobacter pylori (formerly *Campylobacter pylori*)	Gram – curved bacillus	gastritis, stomack ulcers, stomach cancer, can be found in the stomach without evidence of disease
Kerstersia species	Gram – bacillus	rare opportunistic pathogen, a pseudomonad
Kingella species (some formerly *Moraxella* species)	Gram – coccobacillus	uncommon human pathogen
Klebsiella oxytoca	Gram – bacillus	common gut flora, coliform, opportunist
Klebsiella pneumoniae subsp. *ozaenae*	Gram – bacillus	rare cause of infection
Klebsiella pnemoniae subsp. *pneumoniae*	Gram – bacillus	common gut flora, coliform, opportunist
Klebsiella pneumoniae subsp. *rhinoscleromatis*	Gram – bacillus	rare cause of infection
Kluyvera ascorbata (formerly enteric group 8)	Gram – bacillus	rare isolate, coliform
Kluyvera cryocrescens (formerly enteric group 8)	Gram – bacillus	rare isolate, coliform
Kocuria species (some formerly *Micrococcus* species)	Gram + coccus	infections like the coagulase-negative staphylococci but much less common
Kurthia species	Gram + bacillus	rare cause of human infection, mainly animal source
Lactobacillus species	Gram + bacillus	rare cause of human infection, commonly found in normal vaginal flora, some species commonly used in food products
Lactococcus species	Gram + coccus or short bacillus	streptococcus-like, uncommon cause of human infection
Lautropia mirabilis	Gram – coccus	rare isolate
Leclercia adecarboxylata (formerly enteric group 41)	Gram – bacillus	rare isolate, coliform
Legionella anisa	Gram – bacillus	cause of Legionnaire's disease

Legionella feelei	Gram – bacillus	cause of Legionnaire's disease
Legionella micdadei (formerly *Tatlockia*)	Gram – bacillus	cause of Legionnaire's disease
Legionella pneumophila	Gram – bacillus	most common cause of Legionnaire's disease
Leifsonia species (formerly 'C. aquaticum')	Gram + bacillus	rare cause of human infection
Leminorella species (formerly enteric group 57)	Gram – bacillus	rare isolate, coliform
Leptospira species	spirochete, not Gram stained	cause of leptospirosis
Leptotrichia buccalis	Gram – bacillus	anaerobic, part of salivary flora
Leuconostoc species	Gram + coccus or short bacillus	streptococcus-like, uncommon cause of human infection
Listeria monocytogenes	Gram + bacillus	rare maternal and newborn infections, rare infections of compromised hosts
Listeria species (not *monocytogenes*)	Gram + bacillus	rare human infection
Maricaulis species	Gram – bacillus	rare infection, opportunistic, a pseudomonad
Megasphaera species	Gram – coccus	anaerobic, rare cause of infection
Methylobacterium species	Gram – bacillus	rare infection, opportunistic, a pseudomonad
Microbacterium species	Gram + bacillus	rare cause of human infection
Micrococcus species	Gram + coccus	infections like the coagulase-negative staphylococci but much less common
Mobiluncus species	Gram – bacillus, often curved	anaerobic, found in vaginal microflora
Moellerella wisconsensis (formerly enteric group 46)	Gram – bacillus	rare isolate, coliform
Moraxella atlantae	Gram – coccus or bacillus	uncommon isolate
Moraxella catarrhalis (formerly *Neisseria catarrhalis* and *Branhamella catarrhalis*)	Gram – coccus	respiratory infections, often a normal part of oropharyngeal flora
Moraxella lacunata	Gram – coccus or bacillus	uncommon isolate

Moraxella nonliquefaciens	Gram – coccus or bacillus	uncommon isolate
Moraxella osloensis	Gram – coccus or bacillus	uncommon isolate
Morganella subsp. *morganii* (formerly *Proteus morganii*)	Gram – bacillus	urinary tract infections, coliform, opportunist, occasional normal gut flora
Morococcus cerebrosus	Gram – coccus	rare isolate
Mycobacterium abscessus	not Gram stained	uncommon cause of human infection
Mycobacerium asiaticum	not Gram stained	uncommon cause of human infection
Mycobacterium avium	not Gram stained	cause of opportunistic infections
Mycobacterium branderi	not Gram stained	uncommon cause of human infection
Mycobacterium celatum	not Gram stained	uncommon cause of human infection
Mycobacterium chelonae	not Gram stained	uncommon cause of human infection, opportunistic
Mycobacterium conspicuum	not Gram stained	uncommon cause of human infection
Mycobacterium fortuitum	not Gram stained	uncommon cause of human infection, opportunistic
Mycobacterium gastri	not Gram stained	uncommon cause of human infection
Mycobacterium genavense	not Gram stained	uncommon cause of human infection
Mycobacterium gordonae	not Gram stained	uncommon cause of human infection, often a contaminant
Mycobacterium haemophilum	not Gram stained	uncommon cause of human infection, skin and lymph node
Mycobacterium heidelbergense	not Gram stained	uncommon cause of human infection
Mycobacterium interjectum	not Gram stained	uncommon cause of human infection
Mycobacterium intracellulare	not Gram stained	cause of opportunistic infections
Mycobacterium kansasii	not Gram stained	uncommon cause of human infection, opportunistic
Mycobacterium lentiflavum	not Gram stained	uncommon cause of human infection
Mycobacterium leprae	not Gram stained	cause of leprosy
Mycobacterium malmoense	not Gram stained	uncommon cause of human infection, pulmonary
Mycobacterium marinum	not Gram stained	uncommon cause of human infection, skin

Mycobacterium mucogenicum	not Gram stained	uncommon cause of human infection
Mycobacterium scrofulaceum	not Gram stained	uncommon cause of human infection, lymph node
Mycobacterium shimoidei	not Gram stained	uncommon cause of human infection
Mycobacterium simiae	not Gram stained	uncommon cause of human infection
Mycobacterium smegmatis	not Gram stained	uncommon cause of human infection
Mycobacterium szulgai	not Gram stained	uncommon cause of human infection
Mycobacterium terrae	not Gram stained	uncommon cause of human infection
Mycobacterium triplex	not Gram stained	uncommon cause of human infection
Mycobacterium tuberculosis	not Gram stained	cause of tuberculosis
Mycobacterium ulcerans	not Gram stained	uncommon cause of human infection, skin
Mycobacterium xenopi	not Gram stained	uncommon cause of human infection, pulmonary
Mycoplasma buccale	not Gram stained	oral commensal
Mycoplasma faucium	not Gram stained	oral commensal
Mycoplasma fermentans	not Gram stained	urogenital and oral sites, possible cause of sepsis in HIV-infected patients
Mycoplasma genitalium	not Gram stained	genital source, cause of urethral inflammation
Mycoplasma hominis	not Gram stained	urogenital and oral commensal
Mycoplasma lipophilum	not Gram stained	oral commensal
Mycoplasma orale	not Gram stained	oral commensal
Mycoplasma penetrans	not Gram stained	urogenital source, disease causation uncertain
Mycoplasma pirum	not Gram stained	unvalidated cause of AIDS-associated illnesses
Mycoplasma pneumoniae	not Gram stained	common agent of respiratory infection
Mycoplasma primatum	not Gram stained	genital source
Mycoplasma salivarium	not Gram stained	oral commensal
Mycoplasma spermatophilum	not Gram stained	genital source
Myroides species	Gram – bacillus	rare infection, opportunistic, a pseudomonad

(formerly a *Flavobacterium*)

Neisseria animaloris (formerly CDC EF-4)	Gram – coccobacillus	animal bites, rare cause of infection
Neisseria cinerea	Gram – coccus	uncommon cause of infection
Neisseria flavescens	Gram – coccus	uncommon cause of infection, part of salivary flora
Neisseria gonorrhoeae	Gram – coccus	cause of gonorrhea and rare systemic illness, a sexually transmitted disease
Neisseria lactamica	Gram – coccus	uncommon cause of infection, part of salivary flora
Neisseria meningitidis	Gram – coccus	meningitis, blood-borne infection, respiratory infection
Neisseria mucosa	Gram – coccus	uncommon cause of infection, part of salivary flora
Neisseria polysaccharea	Gram – coccus	uncommon cause of infection, part of salivary flora
Neisseria sicca	Gram – coccus	uncommon cause of infection, part of salivary flora
Neisseria subflava	Gram – coccus	uncommon cause of infection, part of salivary flora
Nocardia asteroides	Gram variable	uncommon cause of opportunistic infections
Ochrobactrum species	Gram – bacillus	rare infection, opportunistic, a pseudomonad
Odoribacter species	Gram – bacillus	anaerobic
Oerskovia species	Gram + bacillus	rare cause of human infection
Oligella ureolytica	Gram – coccus or bacillus	rare isolate
Oligella urethralis	Gram – coccus or bacillus	uncommon isolate
Olsenella species	Gram + bacillus	anaerobic, dental source infections
Orientia tsutsugamushi (formerly *Rickettsia tsutsugamushi*)	not Gram stained	cause of scrub typhus
Paenibacillus species	Gram + bacillus	spore-forming, rare cause of human infection
Pandoraea species	Gram – bacillus	rare infection, opportunistic, a pseudomonad
Pantoea species	Gram – bacillus	rare isolate, coliform

(formerly *Enterobacter* species)

Parabacteroides distasonis (formerly *Bacteroides distasonis*)	Gram – bacillus	anaerobic, common bowel flora
Pasteurella multocida	Gram – coccobacillus	animal bites, wounds, rare respiratory pathogen, of animal sources
Pasteurella species (not *multocida*)	Gram – coccobacilllus	rare causes of infection, some species are of animal sources
Pediococcus species	Gram + coccus	infections like the coagulase-negative staphylococci but much less common
Peptococcus species	Gram + coccus	anaerobic, part of bowel flora
Peptoniphilus asaccharolyticus (formerly *Peptostreptococcus asacharolyticus*)	Gram + coccus	anaerobic, associated with infection from bowel and other mucosal sources
Peptostreptococcus anaerobius	Gram + coccus	anaerobic, associated with infection from bowel and other mucosal sources
Pleisiomonas shigelloides	Gram – bacillus	rare isolate, coliform, putative cause of diarrhea
Porphyromonas species (formerly *Bacteroides*)	Gram – bacillus	anaerobic, part of oral and bowel flora
Prevotella species (formerly *Bacteroides*)	Gram – bacillus	anaerobic, part of mucosal flora
Propionibacterium species	Gram + bacillus	rare cause of human infection, commonly found as normal skin and gut flora
Proteus mirabilis	Gram – bacillus	urinary tract infections, coliform, commonly found in gut flora, opportunist
Proteus penneri	Gram – bacillus	uncommon isolate, coliform
Proteus vulgaris	Gram – bacillus	urinary tract infections, coliform, commonly found in gut flora, opportunist
Providencia alcalifaciens	Gram – bacillus	uncommon isolate, coliform
Providenica rettgeri	Gram – bacillus	coliform, occasional gut commensal, opportunist
Providencia rustigianii	Gram – bacillus	uncommon isolate, coliform
Providencia stuartii	Gram – bacillus	coliform, occasional gut commensal, opportunist
Pseudoflavonifractor species (formerly *Bacteroides capillosus*)	Gram – bacillus	anaerobic, uncommon pathogen, part of bowel flora
Pseudomonas aeruginosa	Gram – bacillus	prototype pseudomonad, infection of the

		lung in cystic fibrosis, opportunist, common nosocomial pathogen
Pseudomonas fluorescens	Gram – bacillus	rare opportunist, environmental source
Pseudomonas luteola (formerly *Chryseomonas luteola*)	Gram – bacillus	rare opportunist
Pseudomonas oryzihabitans (formerly *Flavimonas oryzihabitans*)	Gram – bacillus	rare opportunist
Pseudmonas stutzeri	Gram – bacillus	rare opportunist
Psychrobacter immobilis (formerly *Moraxella*)	Gram – coccus or bacillus	uncommon isolate
Psychrobacter phenylpyruvicus (formerly *Moraxella*)	Gram – coccus or bacillus	uncommon isolate
Rahnella species	Gram – bacillus	uncommon isolate, coliform
Ralstonia pickettii (formerly *Burkholderia pickettii* and *Pseudomonas pickettii*)	Gram – bacillus	rare opportunist, a pseudomonad
Rhodococcus equi (formerly *Corynebacterium equi*)	Gram + bacillus	rare opportunist
Rickettsia africae	not Gram stained	cause of African spotted fever
Rickettsia australis	not Gram stained	cause of Queensland tick typhus
Rickettsia conorii	not Gram stained	cause of Mediterranean spotted fever
Rickettsia japonica	not Gram stained	cause of Japanese spotted fever
Rickettsia prowazekii	not Gram stained	cause of epidemic typhus
Rickettsia rickettsii	not Gram stained	cause of Rocky Mountain spotted fever
Rickettsia typhi	not Gram stained	murine typhus
Roseomonas species (formerly known as 'Gram negative pink cocci')	Gram – cocci or bacilli	rare opportunist
Rothia species	Gram variable	rare opportunist
Salmonella enterica	Gram – bacillus	cause of diarrhea and occasional systemic illnesses, many names which appear to be species designations are but serotype names, coliform
Salmonella serotype Paratyphi	Gram – bacillus	causes typhoid fever-like illness, coliform
Salmonella serotype Typhi	Gram – bacillus	cause of typhoid fever, coliform

Schineria species	Gram – bacillus	rare opportunist, a pseudomonad
Selenomonas species	Gram – bacillus	anaerobic, uncommon pathogen
Serratia liquefaciens	Gram – bacillus	uncommon isolate, coliform
Serratia marcescens	Gram – bacillus	occasional component of normal flora, coliform, opportunist especially in hospital settings
Serratia odifera	Gram – bacillus	uncommon isolate, coliform
Serratia plymuthica	Gram – bacillus	uncommon isolate, coliform
Serratia rubidaea	Gram – bacillus	uncommon isolate, coliform
Shewanella species	Gram – bacillus	rare opportunist, a pseudomonad
Shigella boydii	Gram – bacillus	cause of diarrhea, coliform
Shigella dysenteriae	Gram – bacillus	cause of diarrhea and HUS
Shigella flexneri	Gram – bacillus	cause of diarrhea, coliform
Shigella sonnei	Gram – bacillus	cause of diarrhea, coliform
Sphingobacterium species (formerly a *Flavobacterium*)	Gram – bacillus	rare opportunist, a pseudomonad
Sphingomonas species (formerly a *Flavobacterium*)	Gram – bacillus	rare opportunist, a pseudomonad
Spirillum minus	spirochete, poorly Gram staining	rare cause of rat bite fever
Staphylococcus aureus	Gram + coccus	wound, skin, bacteremia, bone, joint, pneumonia, heart, post-surgical, intravenous line, food poisoning
Staphylococcus auricularis	Gram + coccus	one of the coagulase-negative staphylococci, infections of devices and opportunistic infections
Staphylococcus capitis	Gram + coccus	one of the coagulase-negative staphylococci, infections of devices and opportunistic infections
Staphylococcus caprae	Gram + coccus	one of the coagulase-negative staphylococci, infections of devices and opportunistic infections
Staphylcoccus cohnii	Gram + coccus	one of the coagulase-negative staphylococci, infections of devices and opportunistic infections

Staphylococcus epidermidis	Gram + coccus	one of the coagulase-negative staphylococci, infections of devices and opportunistic infections, the most common coagulase-negative staphylococcus causing infection
Staphylococcus haemolyticus	Gram + coccus	one of the coagulase-negative staphylococci, infections of devices and opportunistic infections
Staphylococcus hominis	Gram + coccus	one of the coagulase-negative staphylococci, infections of devices and opportunistic infections
Staphylococcus lugdunensis	Gram + coccus	one of the coagulase-negative staphylococci, infections of devices and opportunistic infections
Staphylococcus saccharolyticus	Gram + coccus	one of the coagulase-negative staphylococci, infections of devices and opportunistic infections
Staphylococcus saprophyticus	Gram + coccus	one of the coagulase-negative staphylococci, infections of devices and opportunistic infections
Staphylococcus schleiferi	Gram + coccus	one of the coagulase-negative staphylococci, infections of devices and opportunistic infections
Staphylococcus simulans	Gram + coccus	one of the coagulase-negative staphylococci, infections of devices and opportunistic infections
Staphylococcus warneri	Gram + coccus	one of the coagulase-negative staphylococci, infections of devices and opportunistic infections
Staphylcoccus xylosus	Gram + coccus	one of the coagulase-negative staphylococci, infections of devices and opportunistic infections
Stenotrophomonas maltophilia (formerly *Xanthomonas maltophilia* and *Pseudomonas maltophilia*)	Gram – bacillus	rare opportunist, a pseudomonad
Stomatococcus species	Gram + coccus	infections like the coagulase-negative staphylococci but much less common
Streptobacillus moniliformis	Gram – bacillus	rare cause of systemic illness, from rodents
Streptococcus agalacticae	Gram + coccus	maternal and newborn infections
Streptococcus alactolyticus	Gram + coccus	a member of the viridans or non-hemolytic streptococci, uncommon cause of human infection but when so, mainly associated with infections related to oral or intestinal

tract sources

Streptococcus anginosus	Gram + coccus	a member of the viridans or non-hemolytic streptococci, uncommon cause of human infection but when so, mainly associated with infections related to oral or intestinal tract sources, some of these may have group A, C, and G streptococcal carbohydrate capsules/antigens
Streptococcus bovis	Gram + coccus	a member of the viridans or non-hemolytic streptococci, uncommon cause of human infection but when so, mainly associated with infections related to oral or intestinal tractsources; occasional blood-borne infections and endocarditis
Streptococcus constellatus	Gram + coccus	a member of the viridans or non-hemolytic streptococci, uncommon cause of human infection but when so, mainly associated with infections related to oral or intestinal tract sources
Streptococcus cricetus	Gram + coccus	a member of the viridans or non-hemolytic streptococci, uncommon cause of human infection but when so, mainly associated with infections related to oral or intestinal tract sources
Streptococcus crista	Gram + coccus	a member of the viridans or non-hemolytic streptococci, uncommon cause of human infection but when so, mainly associated with infections related to oral or intestinal tract sources
Streptococcus downei	Gram + coccus	a member of the viridans or non-hemolytic streptococci, uncommon cause of human infection but when so, mainly associated with infections related to oral or intestinal tract sources
Streptococcus dysgalactiae subsp. *equisimilis*	Gram + coccus	skin and wound infections, other rare infections (group C or G)
Streptococcus equi subsp. *zooepidemicus*	Gram + coccus	rare human infections, mainly a zoonosis (group C)
Streptococcus equinus	Gram + coccus	a member of the viridans or non-hemolytic streptococci, uncommon cause of human infection but when so, mainly associated with infections related to oral or intestinal tract sources
Streptococcus gordonii	Gram + coccus	a member of the viridans or non-hemolytic streptococci, uncommon cause of human infection but when so, mainly associated

with infections related to oral or intestinal tract sources

Streptococcus infantis	Gram + coccus	a member of the viridans or non-hemolytic streptococci, uncommon cause of human infection but when so, mainly associated with infections related to oral or intestinal tract sources
Streptococcus intermedius	Gram + coccus	a member of the viridans or non-hemolytic streptococci, uncommon cause of human infection but when so, mainly associated with infections related to oral or intestinal tract sources
Streptococcus mitis	Gram + coccus	a member of the viridans or non-hemolytic streptococci, uncommon cause of human infection but when so, mainly associated with infections related to oral or intestinal tract sources
Streptococcus mutans	Gram + coccus	a member of the viridans or non-hemolytic streptococci, uncommon cause of human infection but when so, mainly associated with infections related to oral or intestinal tract sources
Streptococcus oralis	Gram + coccus	a member of the viridans or non-hemolytic streptococci, uncommon cause of human infection but when so, mainly associated with infections related to oral or intestinal tract sources
Streptococcus parasanguinus	Gram + coccus	a member of the viridans or non-hemolytic streptococci, uncommon cause of human infection but when so, mainly associated with infections related to oral or intestinal tract sources
Streptococcus peroris	Gram + coccus	a member of the viridans or non-hemolytic streptococci, uncommon cause of human infection but when so, mainly associated with infections related to oral or intestinal tract sources
Streptococcus pneumoniae	Gram + coccus	pneumonia, middle ear infections, sinusitis, meningitis, blood-borne infection
Streptococcus pyogenes	Gram + coccus	strep throat, scarlet fever, skin and wound infections, invasive infection, rheumatic fever, glomerulonephritis
Streptococcus rattus	Gram + coccus	a member of the viridans or non-hemolytic streptococci, uncommon cause of human infection but when so, mainly associated with infections related to oral or intestinal

tract sources

Streptococcus salivarius	Gram + coccus	a member of the viridans or non-hemolytic streptococci, uncommon cause of human infection but when so, mainly associated with infections related to oral or intestinal tract sources
Streptococcus sanguinis	Gram + coccus	a member of the viridans or non-hemolytic streptococci, uncommon cause of human infection but when so, mainly associated with infections related to oral or intestinal tract sources
Streptococcus sobrinus	Gram + coccus	a member of the viridans or non-hemolytic streptococci, uncommon cause of human infection but when so, mainly associated with infections related to oral or intestinal tract sources
Streptococcus vestibularis	Gram + coccus	a member of the viridans or non-hemolytic streptococci, uncommon cause of human infection but when so, mainly associated with infections related to oral or intestinal tract sources
Streptomyces species	Gram variable	uncommon skin infection, rare opportunists
Succinimonas specis	Gram – bacillus	anaerobic, uncommon pathogen
Succinvibrio species	Gram – bacillus or curved bacillus	anaerobic, uncommon pathogen
Sutterella species (formerly *Campylobacter*)	Gram – bacillus	anaerobic, uncommon pathogen
Suttonella indologenes (formerly *Kingella indologenes*)	Gram – coccobacillus	rare cause of infection
Tatumella species	Gram – bacillus	uncommon isolate, coliform
thermophilic actinomycetes	Gram variable	not a cause of infection but associated with hypersensitivity pneumonitis
Trabulsiella species	Gram – bacillus	uncommon isolate, coliform
Treponema pallidum	spirochete, not Gram stained	cause of syphilis
Turicella otitidis	Gram + bacillus	rare cause of human infection
Ureaplasma parvum (formerly a biotype of *Ureaplasma urealyticum*)	not Gram stained	genital commensal
Ureaplasma urealyticum	not Gram stained	genital commensal, possible cause of urethral inflammation, associated with

disorders of newborn and pregnancy

Vagococcus species	Gram + coccus	very rare infections
Veillonella species	Gram – coccus	anaerobic, rare cause of infection
Vibrio alginolyticus	Gram – curved bacillus	uncommon isolate, opportunist
Vibrio cholerae	Gram – curved bacillus	cause of cholera
Vibrio cincinnatiensis	Gram – curved bacillus	uncommon isolate, opportunist
Vibrio damsela	Gram – curved bacillus	uncommon isolate, opportunist
Vibrio fluvialis	Gram – curved bacillus	uncommon isolate, opportunist
Vibrio furnissii	Gram – curved bacillus	uncommon isolate, opportunist
Vibrio harveyi	Gram – curved bacillus	uncommon isolate, opportunist
Vibrio hollisae	Gram – curved bacillus	uncommon isolate, opportunist
Vibrio metschnikovii	Gram – curved bacillus	uncommon isolate, opportunist
Vibrio mimicus	Gram – curved bacillus	uncommon isolate, opportunist
Vibrio parahaemolyticus	Gram – curved bacillus	cause of diarrhea and invasive infection
Vibrio vulnificus	Gram – curved bacillus	uncommon isolate, opportunist
Weeksella virosa	Gram – bacillus	rare opportunist, a pseudomonad
Wolinella species	Gram – bacillus or curved	anaerobic, uncommon pathogen
Yersinia bercovieri	Gram – bacillus	uncommon isolate, coliform
Yersinia enterocolitica	Gram – bacillus	cause of diarrhea and abdominal pain, coliform, rarely invasive
Yersinia frederiksenii	Gram – bacillus	uncommon isolate, coliform
Yersinia intermedia	Gram – bacillus	uncommon isolate, coliform
Yersinia kristensenii	Gram – bacillus	uncommon isolate, coliform
Yersinia mollaretii	Gram – bacillus	uncommon isolate, coliform
Yersinia pestis	Gram – bacillus	cause of plague, a zoonosis
Yersinia pseudotuberculosis	Gram – bacillus	cause of diarrhea and abdominal pain, coliform, rarely invasive
Yersinia rohdei	Gram – bacillus	uncommon isolate, coliform
Yokenella species (formerly enteric group 45)	Gram – bacillus	uncommon isolate, coliform

"Though I am always in haste,
I am never in a hurry."
John Wesley
Letters, December 10, 1777

XX. Index

Clostridium tetani, 50-51, 188, 258, 269
Clotrimazole, 144
Cloxacillin, 141, 143, 151, 157, 229
Coagulase negative staphylococci, 38, 57, 245, 257
Coagulase test, 37
Coccidioides immitis, 19, 41
Coccus, 19, 38, 75, 245
Cohn, 11
Coliform, 59-60, 114, 150, 153, 159, 224, 245
    multi-resistant, 158, 172, 212
Colonization, 7, 244
Colony (of bacteria), 30-31, 78, 245
Colorado tick fever virus, 29
Comamonas species, 269
Commensal, 245
Communicable disease control, 217, 245
Community-acquired infection, 95-96, 245
Complement, 68, 245
Complement fixation test, 81, 83, 245
Congenital infection, 26-27, 245
Conjugation, 152, 245
Conjunctivitis, 79, 245
Conjugate vaccine, 188-189, 192, 246
Contact Isolation, 113-114, 116, 171
Contact Precautions, 113
Contact tracing, 246
Contagion, 246
Coprococcus species, 269
Coronavirus, 27, 111, 238, 256
Corynebacterium species, 38
Corynebacterium accolens, 269
Corynebacterium afermentans, 269
Corynebacterium amycolatum, 269
Corynebacterium auris, 269
Corynebacterium bovis, 269
Corynebacterium confusum, 269
Corynebacterium coyleae, 269
Corynebacterium diphtheriae, 50, 188, 246, 269
Corynebacterium falsenii, 269

Corynebacterium glucuronolyticum, 269
Corynebacterium group F-1, 269
Corynebacterium group G, 269
Corynebacterium jeikeium, 269
Corynebacterium kutscheri, 269
Corynebacterium macginleyi, 269
Corynebacterium matruchotii, 269
Corynebacterium minutissimum, 269
Corynebacterium mucifaciens, 270
Corynebacterium propinquum, 270
Corynebacterium pseudodiphtheriticum, 270
Corynebacterium pseudotuberculosis, 270
Corynebacterium riegelii, 270
Corynebacterium simulans, 270
Corynebacterium singulare, 270
Corynebacterium striatum, 270
Corynebacterium sundvallense, 270
Corynebacterium thomssenii, 270
Corynebacterium ulcerans, 270
Corynebacterium urealyticum, 270
Corynebacterium xerosis, 270
Cost-benefit ratio, 118-119, 246
Cost-effective, 190
Cotrimoxazole, 142, 144
Coxiella burnetii, 255, 270
Coxsackie virus, 29
Creutzfeldt-Jakob Disease (CJD), 47, 94, 137, 196, 199, 224
Cross-infection, 92, 158, 246
Cryptococcus neoformans, 19, 41, 221
Cryptosporidiosis, 219, 246
Cryptosporidium, 19, 43, 45-46, 224, 246
Culture, 73, 77-79, 246
Cupriavidus gilardii, 270
Cupriavidus pauculus, 270
Cytokine, 68, 246
Cytomegalovirus, 26, 91, 144, 198-199
Cytoplasm, 25, 246, 252
Cytotoxin, 50, 246

DATE DUE

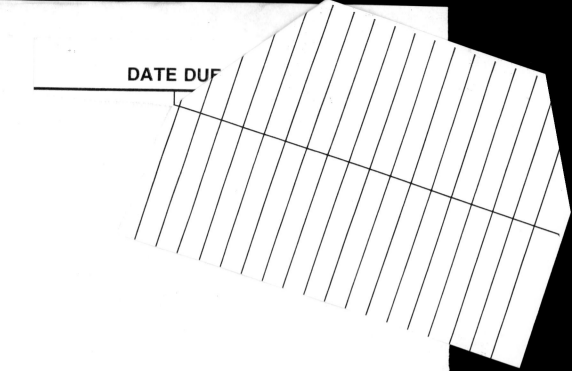

CPSIA information can be obtained at www.ICGtesting.com
Printed in the USA
BVOW05s1501140314

347673BV00007B/64/P